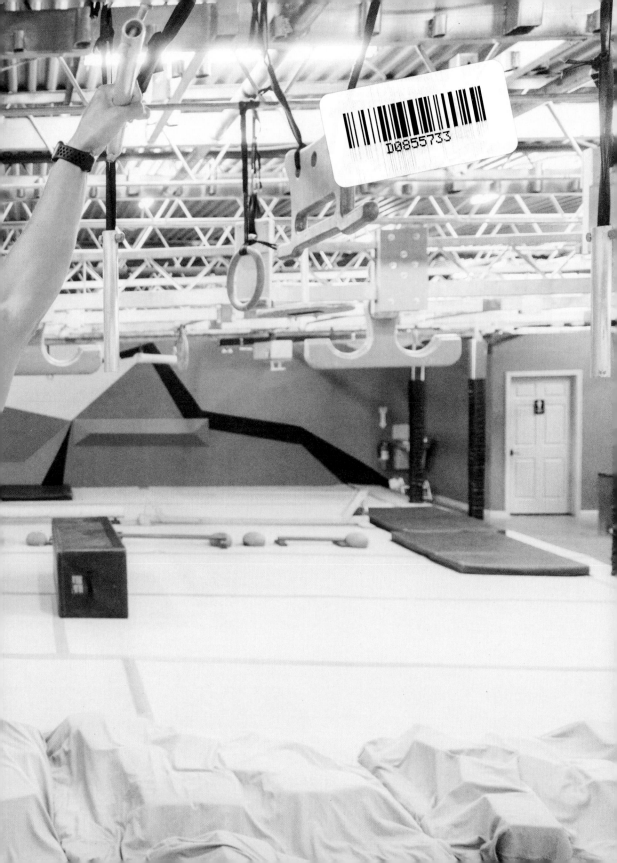

KINGDOM
NINJA

DANIEL
GIL

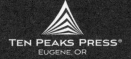
TEN PEAKS PRESS®
EUGENE, OR

Unless otherwise indicated, all Scripture quotations are taken from The ESV® Bible (The Holy Bible, English Standard Version®), copyright © 2001 by Crossway, a publishing ministry of Good News Publishers. Used by permission. All rights reserved.

Scripture quotations marked NLT are taken from the Holy Bible, New Living Translation, copyright © 1996, 2004, 2015 by Tyndale House Foundation. Used by permission of Tyndale House Publishers, Inc., Carol Stream, Illinois 60188. All rights reserved.

Verses marked NIV are taken from the Holy Bible, New International Version®, NIV®. Copyright © 1973, 1978, 1984, 2011 by Biblica, Inc.® Used by permission of Zondervan. All rights reserved worldwide. www.zondervan.com. The "NIV" and "New International Version" are trademarks registered in the United States Patent and Trademark Office by Biblica, Inc.®

Verses marked NKJV are taken from the New King James Version®. Copyright © 1982 by Thomas Nelson, Inc. Used by permission. All rights reserved.

Verses marked AMP are taken from the Amplified® Bible, copyright © 2015 by The Lockman Foundation. Used by permission. (www.Lockman.org)

Published in association with the literary agency of Wolgemuth & Associates

Cover and interior design by Faceout Studio
Photography by Jay Eads

For bulk or special sales, please call 1-800-547-8979.
Email: Customerservice@hhpbooks.com

TEN PEAKS PRESS is a federally registered trademark of the Hawkins Children's LLC. Harvest House Publishers, Inc., is the exclusive licensee of this trademark.

Kingdom Ninja

Copyright © 2023 by Daniel Gil
Published by Ten Peaks Press, an imprint of Harvest House Publishers
Eugene, Oregon 97408

ISBN 978-0-7369-8718-9 (hardcover)
ISBN 978-0-7369-8719-6 (eBook)

Library of Congress Control Number: 2022949320

Printed in Colombia

23 24 25 26 27 28 29 30 31 / NI / 10 9 8 7 6 5 4 3 2 1

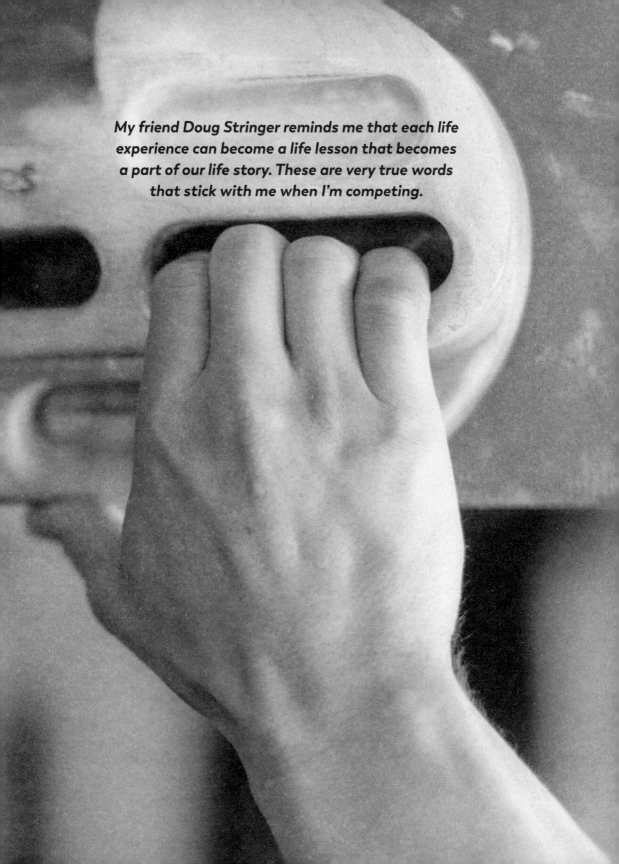

My friend Doug Stringer reminds me that each life experience can become a life lesson that becomes a part of our life story. These are very true words that stick with me when I'm competing.

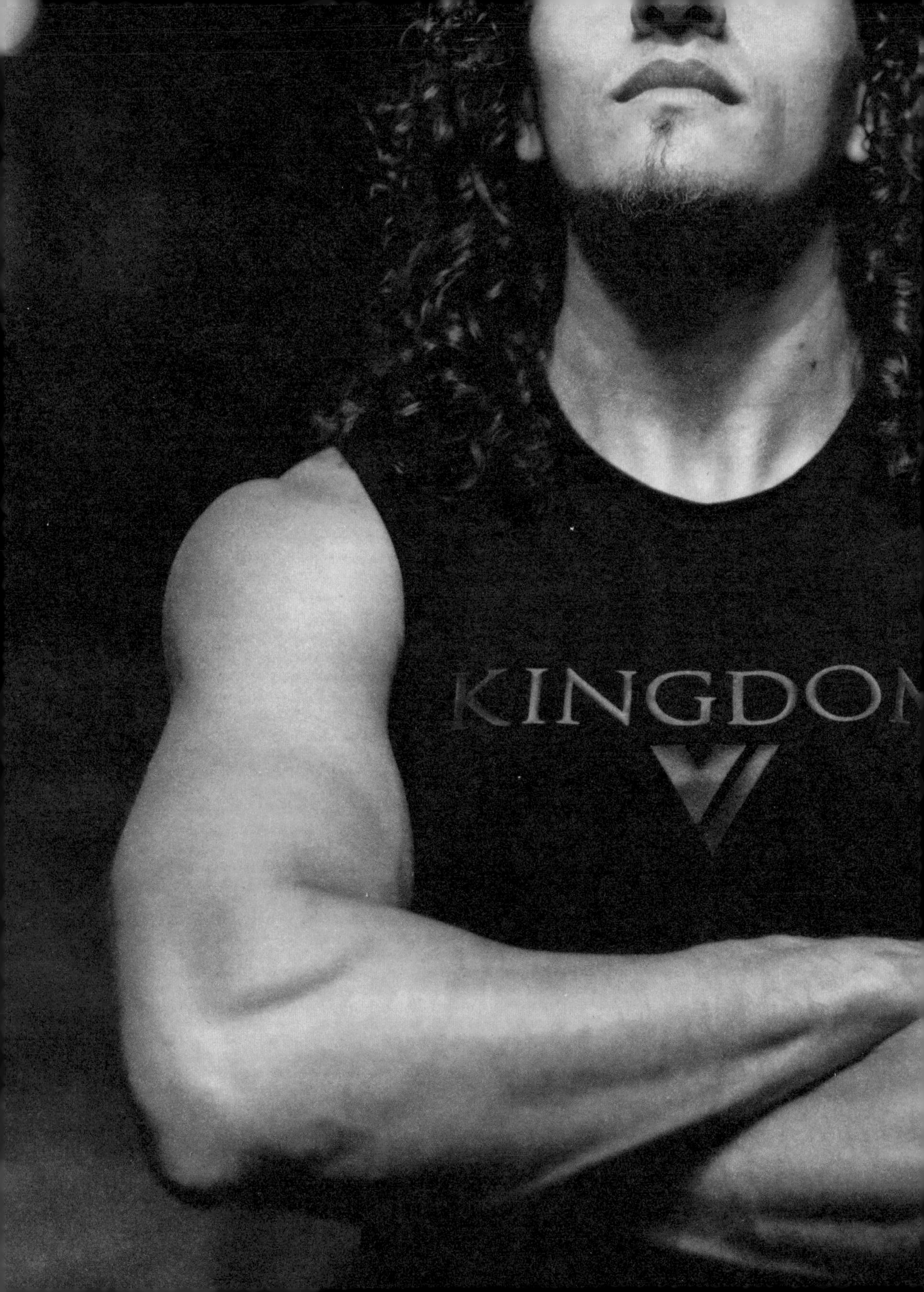
KINGDOM

CONTENTS

Introduction 7

PHYSICAL HEALTH /// 23

1. Body 25
2. Warm-Up 33
3. Workouts 53
4. Ninja OCR Training 65
5. Recovery 91
6. Nutrition 103

MENTAL HEALTH /// 123

7. Wholistic Health 125
8. Motivation 135
9. Mindset 145
10. Giving Back 165

SPIRITUAL HEALTH /// 175

11. A Life of Faith 177
12. Living for Greater Things 211

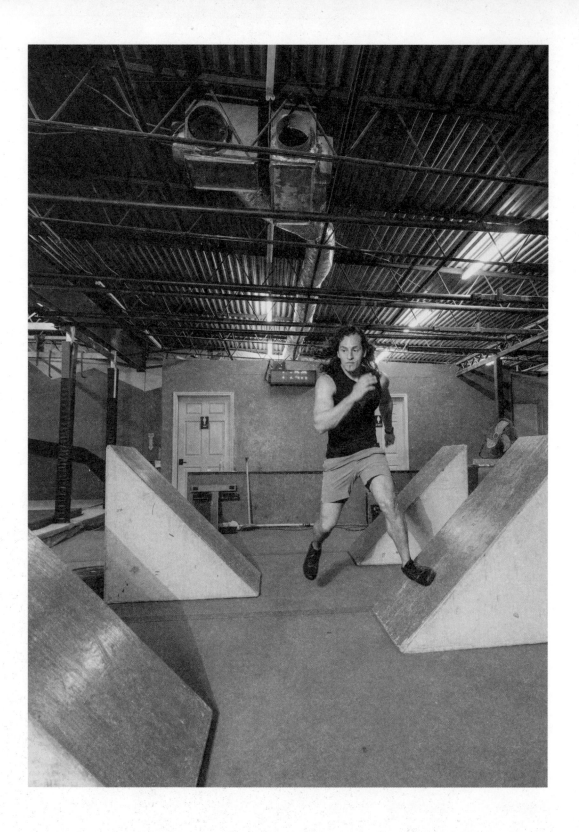

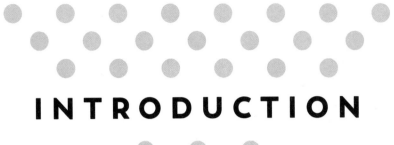

INTRODUCTION

The starting chime rang and we both exploded, flying up the steps as fast as we could. Austin Gray had faster technique (or springs in his legs) and pulled out way ahead, and for a moment, I panicked. This was the final race of the Power Tower Playoffs—the winner would be crowned the *American Ninja Warrior* champion of 2020—so this was the worst time imaginable to fall behind. But it's ingrained in me that nothing's ever over until it's completely over, so once I got to the top of the steps, I ignored the panic and just focused on moving my body faster.

I immediately erased Austin's lead as I slid down the fire pole. Now we were dead even, and we stayed neck and neck through each obstacle, straining our bodies to gain even a millimeter of an advantage. On the final obstacle, I muscled my way through the Falling Shelf quicker than I ever had before, shot through the air past Austin, and hit the buzzer.

My first thought was, "It's over. I don't have to run any more courses today." And then it hit me: "I've just won this season. I finally did it! I am an *American Ninja Warrior* champion!"

Waves of joy and gratitude washed over me. The sense of accomplishment felt surreal, almost as if I were in a dream. The days, weeks, months, and years of training had finally paid off.

We filmed that day for twelve hours. I was exhausted physically and emotionally, and I was ready for bed. We had run multiple courses and Power Tower races and filmed interviews, B-roll footage, and hero shots. My body was at its limit, but I had just accomplished a dream I had been working toward for years.

After descending the tower, I looked around at the Tacoma Dome, where we filmed that entire season. It was completely empty except for the few remaining crew, who were already hard at work tearing everything down. There was no audience that season due to the COVID pandemic. Not even my wife, Abby, or my family were able to attend because of the restrictions in place. It was just me and a few other people in that huge domed stadium. I took some photos, FaceTimed Abby, thanked several producers, and then picked up my trophy and walked a few blocks back to my hotel room. It was a day I will never forget.

With my entire family back home in Houston, I was in a hotel room alone. But even as tired as I was, I couldn't fall asleep—my mind was racing, and my body was still pumped with adrenaline. I relived the entire season over and over again and then went over every season leading up to this moment. I don't think I slept at all that night before getting up for an early flight back home.

Winning was great, but it was the culmination of thousands of habits and choices along the way to become the best possible version of myself. To be the most whole version of who you were meant to be, you need to pursue not just physical health but also mental and spiritual health. Our bodies are important, but who we are on the inside matters just as much or even more so.

This book is a compilation of the different practices I have learned to build into my life to help me be whole. It's not just for people who want to become ninjas or excel at obstacle course racing, although I have included technical advice to help those who do want my best-kept secrets. Anyone can adopt and adapt these principles on their journey to becoming the healthiest version of themselves. You'll find practical how-tos, exercises, recipes, and tutorials, but also some thoughts about health, life, and the soul. Along the way, you'll hear a little bit about my story and how God has done amazing and mind-blowing things in my life, far and above anything I could ever have imagined. I hope you enjoy this book and find something in here to help push you to who God created you to be.

My Ninja Fascination

How did I get into this very peculiar profession in the first place? It's not like they have a college major for ninja training.

I remember being fascinated with actual ninjas growing up. The Teenage Mutant Ninja Turtles were a big thing for me. The characters were sneaky and stealthy, and they worked with tools and swords to beat the bad guys and save the day. What kid wouldn't want to do that? I also loved the ninja Snake Eyes from G.I. Joe . . . and don't even get me started on Naruto the ninja from the Hidden Leaf village! Multiple years in a row I dressed as a ninja for Halloween. I would simply get a costume in a different color and hand down the smaller one to my younger brother. I even experimented with throwing knives into trees—but gave up that goal as quickly as I started because the knife would always clatter off the tree and onto the ground. I didn't have the patience for it or the correct tools for the task. Bottom line, ninjas were a big deal to me during my childhood.

I had two role models growing up. The first was the hero of my faith, Jesus. He was sinless—He never did anything morally wrong—even though He lived in a fallen world. Jesus was perfect even though He was tempted in every way, and He modeled what is possible if we walk through life trusting in our God. Jesus then paid the ultimate sacrifice by taking upon Himself all of our sin, guilt, and shame, and He literally died for us. By dying in our place, He took upon Himself all the punishment of not just me but all of sinful mankind throughout the ages. But after those famous three days in the grave, He rose victorious over sin and death, proving who He was and giving us the opportunity to once again walk with God in close fellowship, as we were originally created to do. This closeness is possible when we put our hope and trust in His finished work of the cross.

My other hero was the Dragon Ball Z character, Goku. He was this cool-looking, fun-loving fighter with a huge appetite. He could fly, perform all kinds of incredible fighting techniques, and eventually win every battle he faced—often with the help of his friends. I wanted to be like this heroic guy who could save his friends and protect his home. No matter how many times he got knocked down, he always managed to get back up and keep going, not to mention that he got stronger after every fight!

Ultimately, I was drawn to Goku's relatability. For a fake character, he seemed incredibly . . . human. He inspired me with his energy, kindness, and caring. He was respectful to others. He took most situations in stride and rarely got overheated by life. But I was most drawn to his genuine concern for the people closest to him.

I wanted to be a hero like Goku, but before I really knew Christ, the idea of being a hero was mostly centered on me. I didn't yet know how to glorify God, so I wanted to glorify myself and be admired by others.

Only after I learned that Christ laid down His life for me to cover my sin could I begin to think about what true sacrifice looked like.

First Steps

In my second year of Bible school, I became aware of Iron Sports gym in Houston. I needed a job because tuition was due in a week. A buddy said, "I have a job at this gym you might be interested in." My initial thought was—*Nah, I'm not a gym type of guy. I've trained my whole life, but I don't lift weights. I do bodyweight stuff. I run. I jump. I climb on things.* But then he said, "No, it's a ninja gym." He didn't have to say another word. I was hooked.

I grew up as an athlete and a fan of ninja competitions on TV. G4 was a network primarily focused on video games, but it occasionally carried other

THE NINJA LIFE

IT'S INCREDIBLE to see how fast the ninja sport has grown. If someone watches an episode and says, "I think I'd like to do that," they actually could try! There are gyms in many cities and most states across the nation. It's skill-based movement. In much the same way that children make up games, the sport of ninja came from a play mentality.

When I was a kid, my friends and I played a game called "spider." We couldn't touch the ground, but we had to make our way around the playground without getting tagged by whoever was "it." We would play for hours on end! With ninja, anyone can start anywhere in this up-and-coming sport. And there are already many different leagues nationwide, from recreational to competitive to elite.

And the sport is so fun, guys. You'll be training for an hour and not even realize time has flown by. Instead, you're focusing on overcoming one more obstacle or perfecting your speed and efficiency on another. There's an excitement to this sport of functional fitness that is less about training to win and more about discovering how much you're capable of learning and growing. People are always available to help, assist, and guide.

Being good at the sport is never a guarantee for getting on the *American Ninja Warrior* (*ANW*) show. Hundreds or thousands of strong individuals audition every year. To be on the show, you need not only skill but also television's X factor, which the show's producers can utilize to reach a certain audience. Every year, some of my friends who audition are in a league of their own in terms of skill and strength, but they don't get the call. Some compete on the show just for the television celebrity status. Others just love to compete. Some want to win money, and still others compete to bring awareness to a cause. The list goes on. Everyone I coach at a ninja gym mentions how much fun this sport is . . . but also how much harder it is than it looks on TV!

With the introduction of *American Ninja Warrior Junior*, thousands of kids now compete in leagues all over the country. Most gyms are built around community and teamwork, and try to keep an ultra-competitive mentality at bay. The sport is only growing, and I can't wait to see where it will be in ten years!

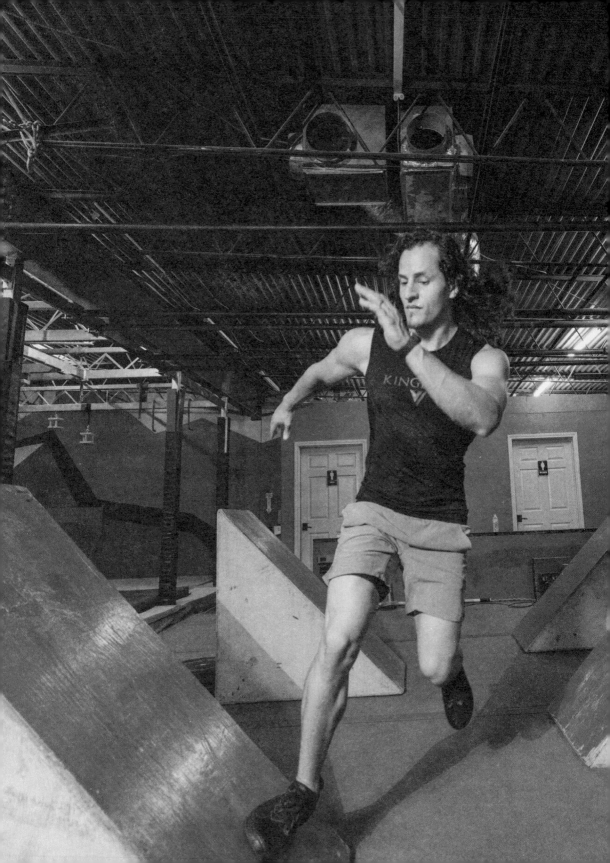

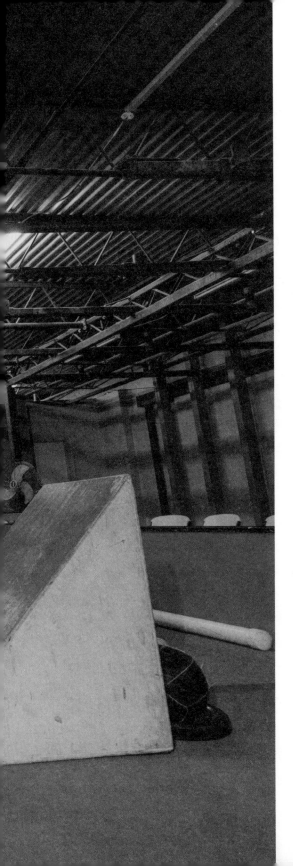

fringe entertainment like UFC and ninja. The original ninja warrior show from Japan, *Sasuke*, was the only show I was allowed to watch on that channel because of its more adult-themed content. I would watch with my brother and three sisters and tell them, "I'm gonna be on that show someday."

I checked out Iron Sports, met the owner, and got to play on some of the obstacles. It was insane. It was part industrial warehouse and part playground. I could have only imagined a place like this in my wildest dreams. The original owner, Sam Sann, built it so he could personally train for ninja competitions. People were running and jumping and climbing all over the place—off ramps, bars, ropes, and all sorts of other obstacles on the ground and hanging from the ceiling. It was like a Rocky gym but for OCR (obstacle course running) and ninja athletes. The people there seemed genuinely joyful and welcoming. People of all ages and sizes and body types were learning to move their bodies around in space and to overcome obstacles and challenges, and they seemed to *love* doing it. This was the kind of stuff I'd always wanted to do.

At the end of my visit, I handed in my résumé and requested a job, but I was told, "We don't have any positions open now, but why don't you get a membership and keep training, and we'll keep you in mind?"

I was discouraged, upset, and in need of a job for tuition money. But at the same time, I was still happy to have found this place and told the Lord I would trust His timing of things and continue to walk by faith.

Another employee, who I did not know, overheard my conversation about wanting a job there. While I was walking to my car, he approached me and said he was about to move to another state but hadn't given his two-weeks' notice yet. He would be willing to train me and just give me his position starting immediately. Miracles do happen!

When I started working there, I was coaching, teaching, cleaning, working at the front desk—the whole nine yards. But also I viewed my job as a ministry, and I tried to say a quick prayer before each class, encourage my students, and be a role model for them.

I still had the pesky problem of tuition for Bible school. I met with the school's financial office and explained that I wouldn't get a check from my new job for a couple of weeks and would not be able to make the tuition deadline. They responded, "We're not allowed to tell you who, but someone has chosen to anonymously come alongside you and take care of your tuition for the entire year." It was like the icing on the cake! Now I had a miracle job *and* miraculous financial provision. I had to pinch myself to make sure I wasn't dreaming!

My response was, *Lord, how can You be so faithful? I'll dedicate these opportunities to You as a thank You!*

Am I in Trouble?

My next step after working at a ninja warrior gym was competing in local competitions around the country. Then I tried to get on the *American Ninja*

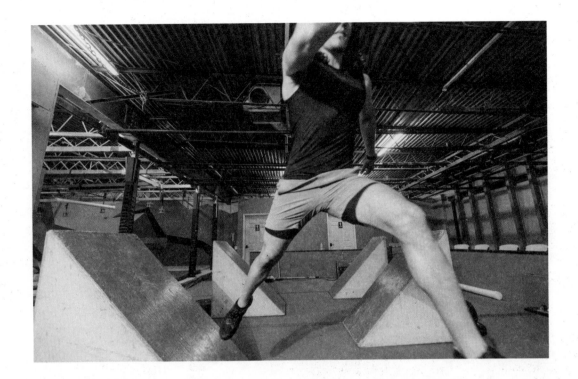

Warrior show itself. Unfortunately, applicants had to be twenty-one, and I was a few days too young. I sent in an audition video anyway . . . to no avail. But I was old enough to be a course tester for the individual obstacles and even do some full course runs. I jumped at the opportunity to showcase my skills and abilities and make some cool new friends and connections.

After a while, some of the producers approached me and said, "Hey, you!" They didn't even know my name! "Come over here, we need to talk."

My immediate thought was, *Oh no, did I break something? Am I in trouble?* (Isn't it amazing how our minds always go to the worst-case scenario first?)

But they basically said, "You're running through these courses so quickly and making them look so easy, we need to adjust the obstacles and make them harder. Who *are* you? Why aren't you a competitor?"

I was blown away! I got myself noticed!

This is my chance . . . don't mess it up! I introduced myself and told them I was too young to compete. And the producers—keep in mind, this is their

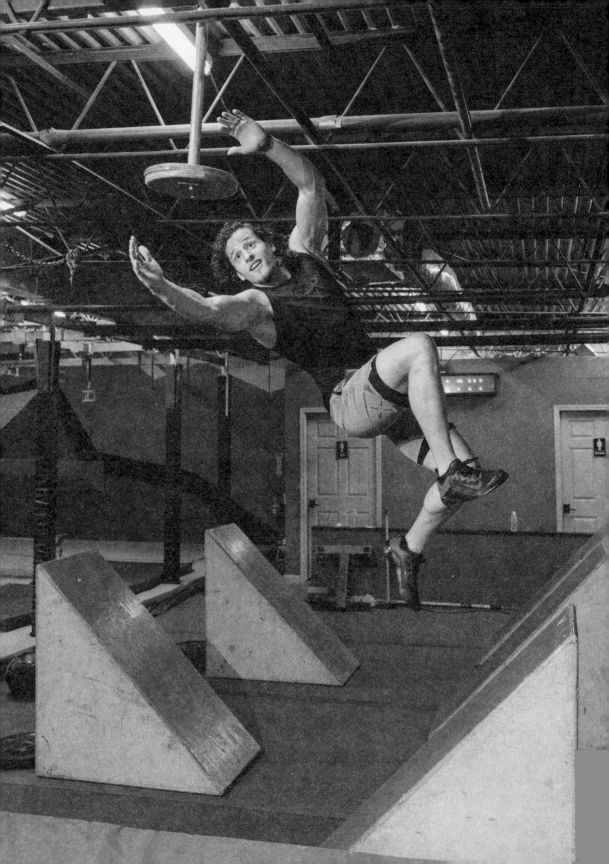

show, but they aren't directly over casting protocols—asked, "How old do you have to be to compete?"

And I said, "Twenty-one."

Then they said they liked me and told me that if I could make it out to Vegas that year, I could test-run the courses at the National Finals as well. They said they wanted to see me compete next year when I was old enough. So I got a ticket, stayed with some friends who were also in town, and got to test stages one to three on season 6 of *American Ninja Warrior*.

Viva Las Vegas

Vegas was . . . well, Vegas. It was hot. Loud. Disorienting. Crowded. But so exciting because I was on an adventure that would take me one step closer to my dream of competing.

I had never been to Vegas before and only had movies as a reference. Honestly, the place was kind of tacky . . . but in an awesome way.

It was up to 118 degrees during the day—much different from the humid heat I was used to in Texas. It's so hot and dry there that they spray water on the ground to keep the dust from being unbearable. They had air conditioning units on top of *other* air conditioning units to keep things cool while filming outside. People wore sunglasses and hats, long sleeves to keep their skin out of direct sunlight, and dust masks to keep their throats clear from the sand. And whatever you do, don't touch *anything* metal that's been under the sun! Because of the heat, and to control audience size and have the ideal lighting that makes the show really pop on TV, they tape from around 8:30 p.m. (or once the sun is completely down) to 4:00 a.m. or even sometimes 5:00 a.m., when the sun comes up and they *have* to stop!

I witnessed how they built these courses out in the desert with things suspended from elaborate scaffolds and with all the lights and sounds of the Las Vegas strip in the background. For a person to succeed there, they would have to be *very* good at focusing and blocking out distractions. But ultimately, these courses were still similar to the courses back at the Iron Sports gym. Ramps. Ropes. Even as a tester, I felt like I was at home on the courses, and I ran and jumped my way through them relatively easily.

Lord, I Trust You . . . but What's Going On?

The next year I made my first *official* video at an eligible age, and I felt great about it. I filled out the incredibly long online application, added the two headshot photos and then . . . waited.

The waiting can be the most difficult part for people because that's when your season can end before it even begins. It can take up to a couple of months for callbacks to begin.

I soon started to hear about many of my friends receiving callbacks from the show. Some of the people who received calls were people I had trained—some of them for just a few weeks before they applied for the show. Yet still no call for me. And so I waited. And waited.

I remember thinking, *Lord, I trust You . . . but what's going on?* I should have been a shoo-in for the show. I had met a few of the producers already. I even made something of a name for myself on the ninja scene as a capable tester the year prior. But . . . I never got the call I was hoping and praying for.

My heart was broken. But even in my prayers of confusion, I didn't lose hope or heart. Instead, I remembered hearing about the famed walk-on line for *ANW* and decided that if that was my last chance for this season, I would do everything in my own power to make it happen and trust God with the results. I tell myself daily, *I will work hard, do my best, and let God take care of the rest*. That's the mentality I chose to have for that moment.

Once *ANW* announces when and where they will film a season, people can go to the locations in advance and form a line for the opportunity to run the course. Before they developed the lottery system for season 11, the producers would select ten or fifteen people from near the front of the line to be official competitors. But how long you might wait could vary based on how early people wanted to show up and unofficially begin the line. I've heard horror stories of friends who waited in line for upwards of three weeks! People will wait in line for hours for a new phone, game, theme-park ride, or even Black Friday . . . but few people can sacrifice the time that these walk-on lines may require. Many would take sleeping bags and stay there the whole time. Not my kind of adventure at all.

My walk-on attempt was in my hometown of Houston. I showed up several hours earlier than the allowed start time, but to my shock and amazement I was still number twenty-seven in line. According to the numbers, I would not even get a chance to run. But I had no other options, so I decided to wait and hope.

As the days inched by, I was hot, sunburned, discouraged, and dehydrated. My only solace was that the competition was on private property at the Berry Center, so we had to vacate each night. Our places in line were recorded, and we got back in line (in the same order) the next morning.

I waited for almost a week. At this point I was feeling a little ridiculous, to be honest. I mean, how many grown men wait in a line, in the sun, for a week, for something that probably isn't going to happen and might not even lead to anything if it does? Some of my family and friends tried to prepare me for the disappointment.

Finally, one afternoon, while sitting in a lawn chair in the middle of the parking lot line that fifty of us had formed, I began to pray. Not a happy prayer either. It was one of frustration, anger, and sadness at my current situation. You see, I had made a promise that I would never hide my feelings from the Lord (as if He didn't already know them). After getting it all off my chest, I ended my prayer by saying that I still trusted Him and that if this didn't work out, I would just try again next year.

Immediately after that prayer I heard a voice from behind me say, "Daniel?" I turned around, and it was one of the producers I'd met before. He said, "What in the world are you doing in this line?"

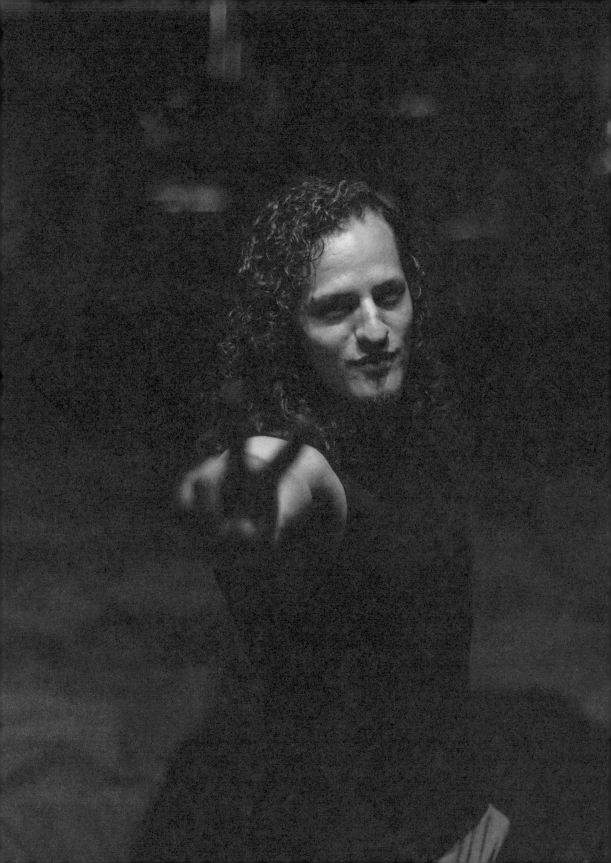

I said, "My audition video wasn't accepted, but I really want to compete. It's on my heart and I know I'm ready." He said they'd received a massive number of videos—thousands that year—and mine must have fallen through the cracks. He said, "Well . . . I'm sorry."

I said, "Me too! Is there anything we can do?"

He asked me my number, and I told him.

"Oh."

He knew what that meant. It meant there was no way I was going to touch the course, since selection was usually on a first-come, first-served basis. Under normal circumstances at least. But then he said, "I want you to go back to your line and wait. And when competition night comes and we send the others away except for a few, I will make sure you get a chance to run the course." And just like that, the conversation was over, and I walked back to my chair.

Finally, the time came. I was nervous and scared, but I could feel the Lord's hand on me the whole way. The sun started setting, the bleachers were filling with audience members, the producer dismantled the walk-on line, and just as he said, he pulled me aside and put me into the competitor's group. Several of the guys asked, "Who is this kid and why is he here?" because I was ushered to the front of the line to check in, register, take my photos, and get my run number!

Typically, walk-ons are thrown to the wolves and made to go first, kind of like human guinea pigs. But I was given an ideal slot a little later, closer to the midnight lunch break, which meant I had time to get mentally prepared and watch a bunch of other guys go through first.

That event, the Houston city qualifiers, was my first opportunity to compete, and I had the fastest time of the entire event that night. What a way to start!

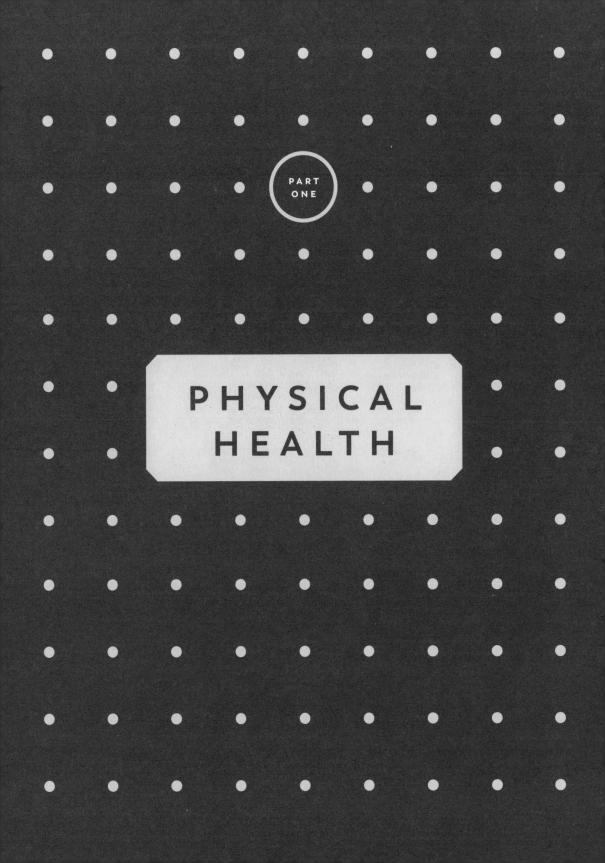

PART
ONE

PHYSICAL HEALTH

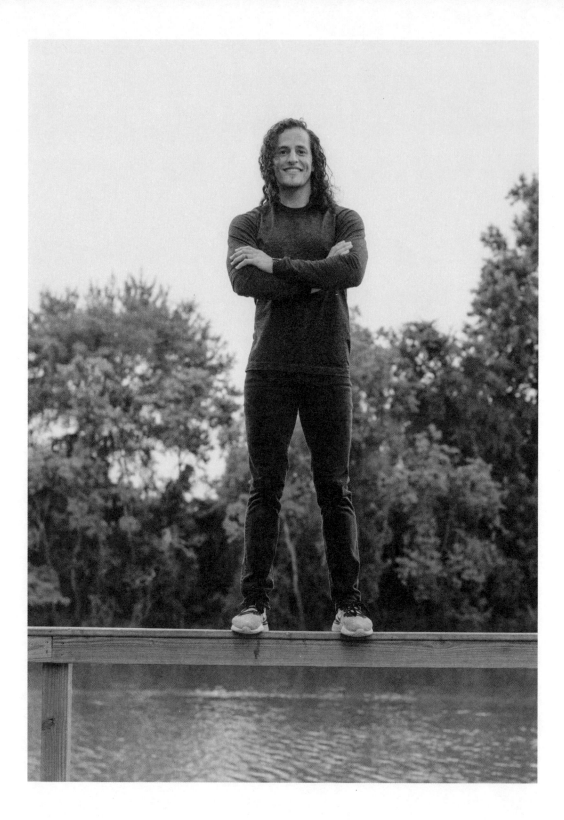

1

BODY

'll never forget when I was in middle school and found out I was obese for my age. I weighed about 155 pounds at twelve years old, which isn't that much less than I weigh now. After being the skinny, athletic monkey of a kid most of my childhood, I had taken a season off from sports and got sucked into a sedentary lifestyle of video games and junk food. All it took was a few months of that, coupled with puberty, and *boom*—recipe for disaster! I was miserable and desperately in need of a change.

Just before I started high school, my dad got a Bowflex home gym. I was so excited because I had seen the commercials and thought, *Oh my gosh, I want a Bowflex body!* I trained on the Bowflex every day. I wanted to be physically capable of doing anything I wanted or needed to do. I got back into soccer for another two seasons and was finally back on track, entering high school fit and healthy and grateful to have learned a valuable life lesson. I would never repeat that mistake again.

In fact, now I work on not being overly obsessive with health. It's about keeping perspective. I don't take care of my body just as an athlete—I take care of it because I want to be physically strong and capable of doing whatever God might call me to do next. Our bodies are gifts from God, gifts we must steward well so we don't waste what we're given.

I don't want to put too much garbage into my body and end up with the type of health problems I see in the world so often. Our bodies are the most incredible machines on the planet. They might *function* on any kind of fuel, but they will only *excel* on the right kind of fuel.

However, there's a way to take all of this too far and be so health-focused that we become unhealthy. I know a lot of people who are enslaved to their diet and exercise regimen. Again, in my opinion, the key is in finding balance. I like chocolate and ice cream a lot. I'm going to enjoy life. I'm going to be a happy athlete and enjoy my rest days and my cheat days. But my normal diet consists of real foods.

There's one piece of advice my dad has always told me. I've seen him as a very strong, very strict, very disciplined man . . . but he has always told me to enjoy life. My dad is full of discipline, but he places a high value on enjoying what he's doing. He's always saying, "Enjoy life. Enjoy it, Daniel! Make the most of it. Don't have regret. Leave things where they lie."

Move Your Body

The first key to fitness is just moving your body. You can't get stronger and faster by sitting on the couch.

I was always the monkey child in my family. I climbed on everything. I loved to move. I was an athlete, and I played almost every sport: baseball, basketball, tennis, roller hockey, even competitive dodgeball! But soccer was the sport I played the most. My dad was a professional soccer player in Colombia and came to the United States on a scholarship to play for Houston Baptist University, which is where he met my mother.

I played soccer off and on my entire childhood, but sad to say, I was never very good! I didn't have the stamina for offense, the drive for defense, or the skills to be a midfielder. But it taught me a lot about hard work, discipline, and teamwork. I'm super competitive (for better and for worse), and even though I was a shy kid and didn't like attention, it was hard for me to be anything but the star player. After a time, I thought, *What am I even doing here?*

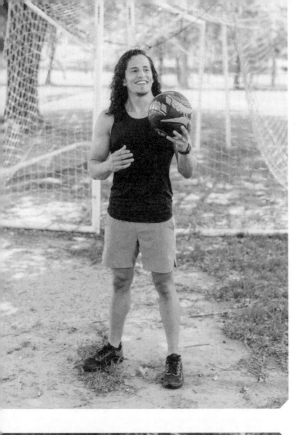

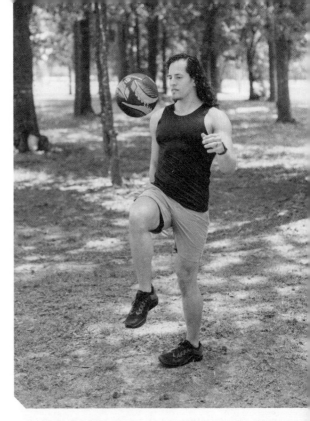

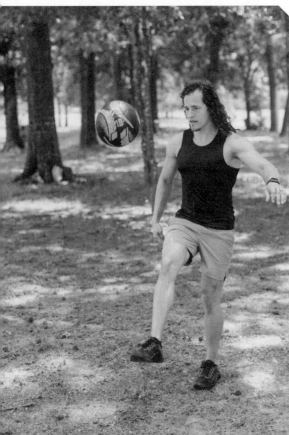

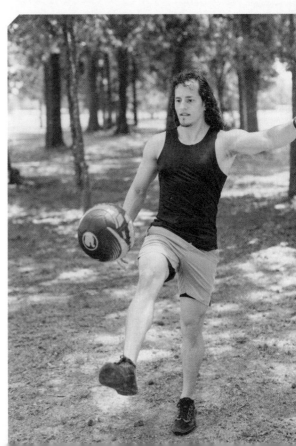

DANCING

During high school I found a new passion for theater, dance, and performing arts. All the dance choreography was really intense. The guys were throwing the girls up in the air and doing backflips, handstand walks, and things like that. Our choreographer would get her inspiration from watching *Dancing with the Stars*, and we'd practice so hard to learn how to do similar moves! This was where I really began to come alive in the spotlight and focus my athleticism into acrobatic feats, and I fell in love with performing.

If traditional sports aren't your thing, maybe put on some music and just move to the beat. You'd be surprised how great a workout it really is.

But I loved the *movements* in soccer and how the athleticism of that sport translates so well to everyday life. The natural cardiovascular fitness you develop in the sport, the core strength, and the agility all lend themselves well to ninja training. After coaching in ninja for about a decade now, I've noticed that soccer players, gymnasts, swimmers, rock climbers, and parkour athletes tend to be the best athletes who come into the ninja gym. You can build a great deal of functional strength and conditioning when playing those sports.

If you are just beginning to improve your fitness, you'll want to prioritize movement to support a healthy heart rate and good blood flow. Start right where you are and find something you like to do that gets you moving. Then set goals and realistic daily steps to work toward those goals. You don't have to be a professional athlete to live a healthier, happier life and achieve greater physical abilities and endurance. You could try taking a regular walk, jogging, riding a bike, or participating in an athletic sport. Routine will be key, and adding movement to your weekly schedule will be a game changer. Personally, I try to move every single day, even on my rest days.

Focus on functionality. It's about building up the muscles and joints for everyday movements: climbing stairs, carrying boxes, getting out of chairs, lifting your children and grandchildren. We all want to be able to do these things for years to come. But unfortunately, far too many people spend the majority of their day sedentary—sitting in a classroom, sitting behind a work desk, or sitting on the couch at home. I'm talking about kids and adults alike. You can build small, brief, daily and weekly habits, but it begins by recognizing and taking ownership of your health. Just take it one day at a time.

The good news is that it's never too late to start moving and taking that first step in your growth. The goal is improvement, and the process is the adventure. And it all starts here.

Consistency

The best ninja athletes aren't necessarily the strongest, but they're the most *consistent*. They're the ones who can regularly perform really well on obstacles on the first try. And they maintain that status, sometimes for years. You could have all the strength in the world and still not be great at constancy . . . yet. For me as a Christian, the greatest legacy and ministry I could leave on this earth is a life of consistency in my walk of faith. That's what I strive for, and that desire also manifests in other areas of my life, like ninja. I will always work hard, always get back up, and always move forward. I work hard to maintain consistency in my life passions.

One of the best things you can do to help build consistency is find a workout partner. Community is life! Build a routine together around any of your health and fitness goals. We are creatures of habit and routine. When you can build a new healthy habit and create a routine that includes it on a regular basis, then you're on your way to becoming a happier, healthier person.

Injury History

I've had lots of injuries during my time as a ninja athlete. The list includes shoulders, arms, wrist, multiple finger tendons, knees, and a broken nose.

Many of my injuries were due to overuse and were completely preventable if I had known then what I know now. Others were just freak accidents that happened in the heat of the moment, much like they do in other sports. Ninja is a very dynamic, aggressive, and high-impact sport. Thankfully though, I've been able to avoid surgery for all of my injuries thus far. (I'm praying it stays that way the rest of my life!) I just have to do a lot of rehab. For example, people can tweak or seriously injure their ankles, knees, or Achilles tendons on the warped wall if the challenges are not attempted properly, *especially* by beginners. Finger tendons are also a huge issue for people who aren't used to aggressively carrying their full body weight like you do in ninja.

I've had multiple partial tears of pulley tendons in my fingers. Often this is due to overtraining . . . or doing a stupid move or taking on a dare without warming up.

Several years ago I destroyed my wrist jumping full speed into a spinning doorknob type of obstacle during a speed course in Dallas. Imagine monkey bars, but with spinning orbs connected to the side. I jumped to grab onto these spinning orbs, with all my weight, at high speed. The orbs spun way faster than I anticipated, and *crunch*—there went something in my wrist. It's been years since the injury, and I still deal with it on occasion. Another time, I decided to start running more for increased cardio. I went way too hard, way too fast, for way too long. Afterward, I couldn't put my full weight on my knee for weeks because of a partial tear. Avoidable.

I've had several partial tears in both shoulders as well. I once had an MRI done on my "good" shoulder when it started to give me issues, only to discover I had two partial tears and a cyst underneath in an avascular (non-blood-flowing) place. It was at that point I really, *really* had to up my physical therapy and rehab game—but also my "prehab" game became a key component to my regular training. There was no other option if I wanted to continue doing what I loved at the level I was doing it, and on the national stage.

STRENGTHS AND WEAKNESSES

I often tell my students (and myself) that finding a weakness in your abilities is not a reason to shrink back in that area, or whine and complain, or avoid it altogether for fear of failure. Instead, look at weakness as an opportunity to grow in an area where you obviously need improvement, and use discipline to overcome the obstacle.

This outlook on life applies to you not only physically but also mentally and even spiritually. You can benefit in all areas of life by realizing that weaknesses don't have to stay weaknesses forever. They don't have to define you. It might take time. It *will* take work. But it is *always* worth it. The pursuit of greatness is itself great.

Upper body mobility became a high priority to me. I now have all sorts of bands and tools I use daily to help my injured or problem areas more fully recover and regain their original strength. I'll explain those exercises and movements in more detail starting on page 91.

More recently, I gashed a chunk out of my nose when I fell on a balance obstacle—a balance obstacle! I'm great at balance obstacles and rarely mess those up thanks to years of soccer and dance. But accidents happen, and unfortunately for my face, *that* scar is a noticeable one.

When I asked my buddy Mike Cook for prayer in recovery (he's had his own facial injuries), he jokingly told me that my face was too pretty and I *needed* a cool scar to look more manly! Unbelievable! The worst part was that the fall itself didn't even hurt that bad; it just removed a lot of skin and couldn't be stitched up that well. Vanity is something Abby (my wife) and Mike are helping me work through. Thankfully, I've since healed up really well without PTSD on my balance game.

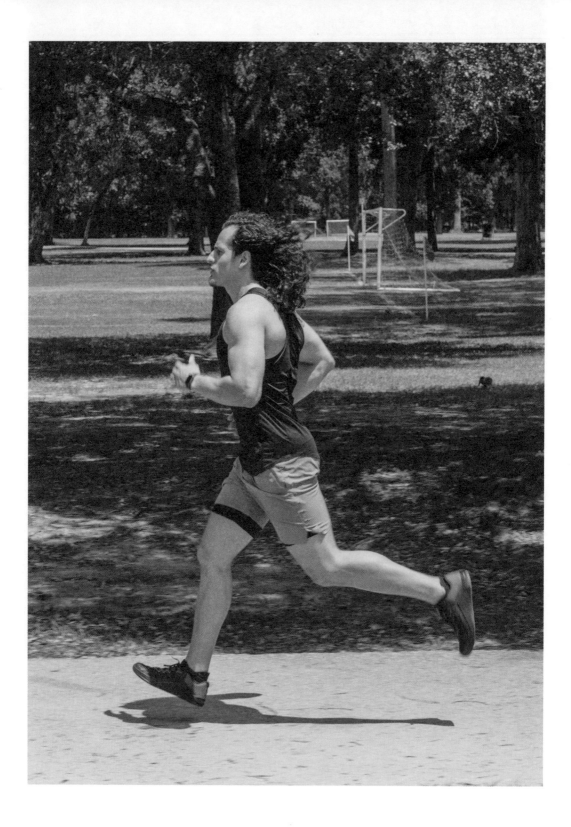

2

WARM-UP

Before starting a workout, it's necessary to have a focused, dynamic warm-up. Every time I have tweaked, twisted, or pulled something during my workouts or competitions, I can always trace it back to a lack of warming up properly. So now, whether in training or competition, I make a high priority of setting aside the time to warm up.

Ninja OCR is a very high-impact sport, and our bodies need to be ready for anything. A proper warm-up gets me feeling primed and ready to tackle my workouts to the fullest. I always give myself at least fifteen to twenty minutes for my warm-up.

+ I jog a mile to work up a sweat and get the blood pumping to my extremities.

+ For about five to ten minutes, I work from lower body to upper body, doing different dynamic stretches and band work to mimic anything I might do during my training that day.

+ I do some light exercises to focus heavily on any past areas of injury so I don't reinjure myself in any way.

+ Be sure to stretch and warm-up equally on both sides of the body.

Dynamic Movements and Stretches

JUMPING JACKS: This is an old school, total-body warm-up exercise.

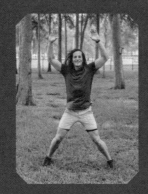

WALKING KNEE HUGS: Much like they sound, just take a step forward, raise your knee to your chest, and grab it. This movement is meant to engage stabilizers, improve balance, and warm up the hamstrings and glutes.

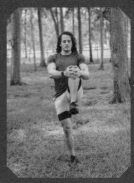

ARM CIRCLES: In any kind of ninja workout, or even for boxers or any athletes using the upper body, it's critical to warm up our delts, traps, and shoulder area. Hold your arms out to your side and circle them. Then repeat, holding them out straight to the front, and then above your head.

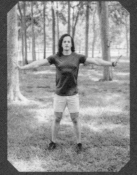

BACKPEDALING: Feet about shoulder-width apart, taking care to not get your chest too far forward, pump your arms and run backward. Start slow so you don't lose balance.

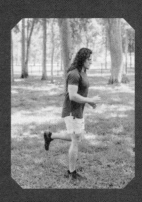

LUNGES: These are essential for any athlete who runs, jumps, or explodes. Great for balance, core, and stabilizer muscles, as well as warming up and strengthening the glutes, quadriceps, and hamstrings. Keeping your chest up, take a large step forward with deep knee bends, then stand up straight. Repeat.

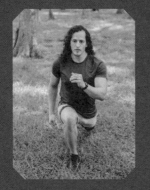

SQUATS: Start with your feet shoulder width apart. Bend your knees to a 90-degree angle, like you're about to sit in a chair, keeping your chest up. Make sure your knees aren't moving past your toes. Then, pushing through your heels, stand up. Repeat.

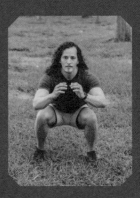

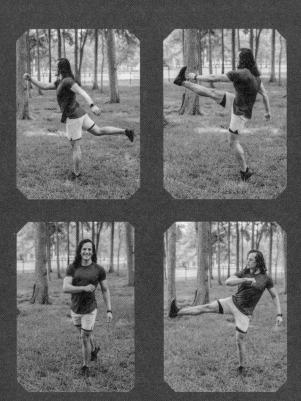

LEG SWINGS: I love this one as a way to warm up my hip socket and lower abdominal area. Grab a bar or the wall for stability (if you need it), and swing your leg front to back, keeping the leg straight. Then swing it side to side.

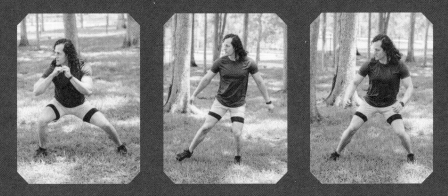

SIDE SHUFFLES: Side shuffles engage the quads, glutes, and calves. Start with your feet about shoulder width apart, lower your butt down and keep your eyes up and your back straight in a good athletic position, and shuffle to the side, taking care not to cross your feet.

Shoulder stretches

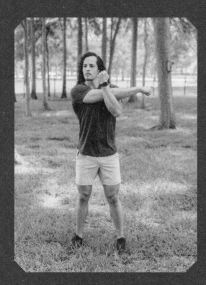
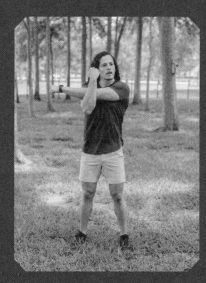

CROSS-BODY SHOULDER STRETCH: While standing, bring your arm horizontally across your chest and use your other arm to pull it toward your chest. Hold a few seconds or until desired. Repeat on the other side.

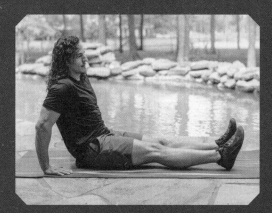
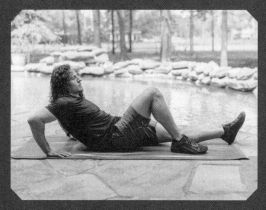

SEATED SHOULDER STRETCH: While seated on the ground, place your hands flat on the ground beside your hips, fingers pointing toward your toes. Don't let them move. Next, slide your legs and bottom forward (without moving your hands) and bend your elbows to lean back. You will instantly feel the stretch in your shoulders. Gently rock side to side to activate a deeper stretch.

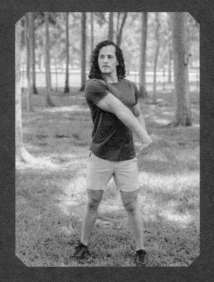

WRIST AND FOREARM STRETCH: Reach one arm out in front of you with palm facing away and fingers pointing downward. Use your other hand to grab your fingers and pull them toward your body. Increase the stretch by then pulling your arm diagonally across your body like a seatbelt. Hold a few seconds or as long as desired. Do the same with the other hand.

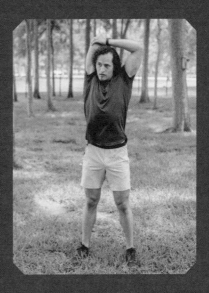

TRICEP STRETCH: Reach your hand straight up. Bending your arm at the elbow, reach your hand behind your head and crawl your hand down the center of your back. Use your other hand to gently pull your elbow toward your head to assist the stretch. Hold for a few seconds or as desired. Do the same with the other arm.

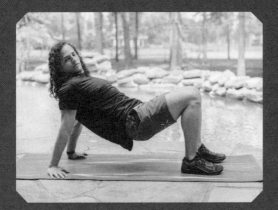

SEATED BICEP STRETCH: While seated on the ground, plant both hands on the ground beside your hips, fingers slightly flared away from your body. Next, bring one and then both feet flat on the ground with knees going upward. Lock your elbows and lift your bottom up. You should immediately begin feeling a deep stretch in both biceps.

Wrist stretches

While on your hands and knees, place your hands flat on the ground and spread your fingers wide. While keeping your elbows locked, turn your shoulders outward and gently begin rocking side to side to stretch the forearms of both arms simultaneously. Maintain for as long as desired. Next, flip your hands over and gently place the tops of your hands against the ground with your fingers pointing in toward each other. Gently apply pressure as you rock side to side. Rotate your wrists so your fingers face toward you, and repeat. Continue as long as desired.

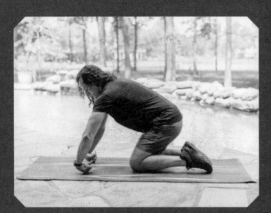 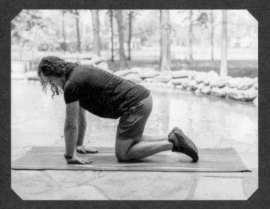

Light Exercises for Warm-Up

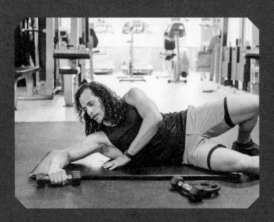 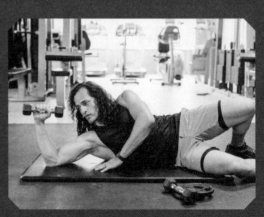

SHOULDER REHAB, WEIGHTED: While lying on your side, propped up on an elbow, hold a one- to five-pound weight in your non-supporting hand, straight up in the air. Slowly lower the weight down toward the ground, engaging the shoulder throughout the motion.

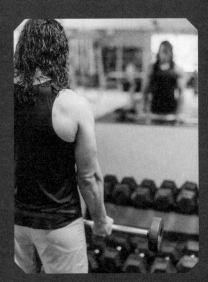
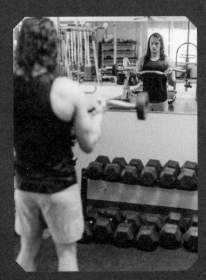

BICEP CURLS: Biceps are an important part of any ninja or OCR athlete's approach, due to their importance in hanging and climbing. Grab a light bar, and with your hands shoulder width apart and palms facing upward, curl the weight upward, squeezing the bicep at the top. You can also do this with a resistance band by stepping on one end of the band and grasping and pulling up the other end.

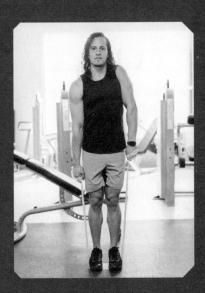
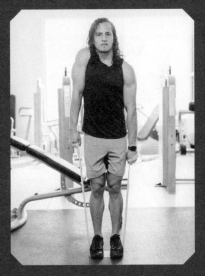

SHOULDER SHRUGS: While holding and stepping on a long resistance band, stand with your feet shoulder width apart, and shrug your shoulders one at a time. This will warm up and activate your shoulders in general and specifically your trapezius muscles.

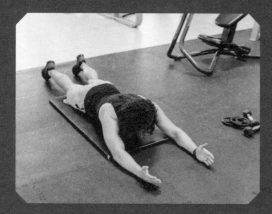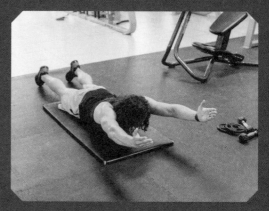

I, Y, T, W: Lying on your stomach, reach both arms out in front of you, making an "I" with your body. Rotate your palms to face upward. Engaging your shoulder and upper back, raise your arms high above your head and then lower them back down.

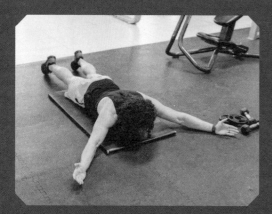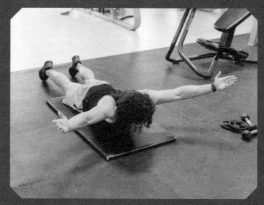

Next, move your arms farther out to form a "Y," raise them up, and lower them down again.

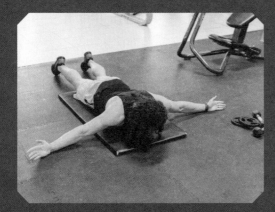
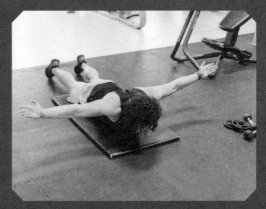

Then move them straight out to the sides to make a "T" and move them up and down.

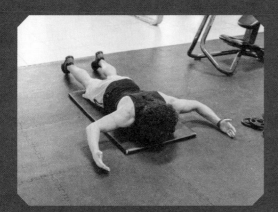
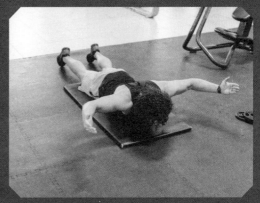

Finally, bring your elbows down toward your hips and bring your hands up toward shoulders, creating a "W" shape, and raise your hands up and down. Complete five to ten sets of each position to really warm up or rehab the shoulders.

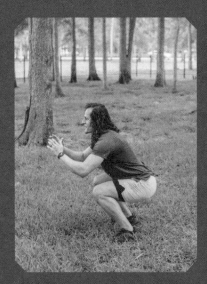
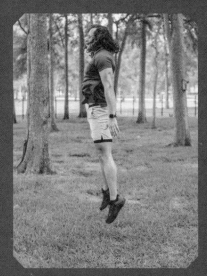

SQUAT JUMPS: Begin with your feet shoulder width apart, squat to 90 degrees, and then jump straight up in the air. This is great for quads, glutes, and calves, and it can also be a cardio movement if done repeatedly.

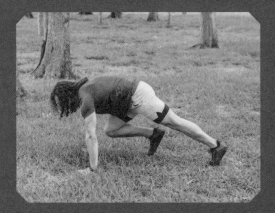
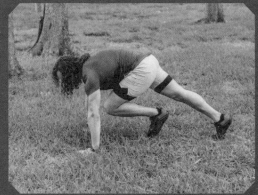

MOUNTAIN CLIMBERS: Begin by getting into a high plank position with your hands shoulder-width apart beneath you. Bring your knee up to your abdomen, keeping your knee directly between your torso and the ground. Alternate legs in a climbing motion.

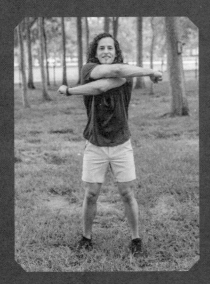 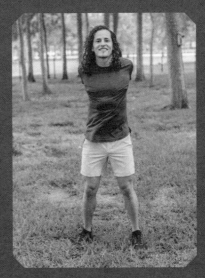

DYNAMIC ARM SWINGS: Standing upright, swing your arms forward and backward, focusing on stretching and loosening up the shoulders. Try clapping your hands both in front of and behind your back while doing this dynamic stretch. Then swing your arms up and down, aiming to get your arms to swing above your shoulders and behind your ears all in one motion, but do not move the arms in a complete circle. Try to go a little bit further with each swing as you loosen and warm up your shoulders.

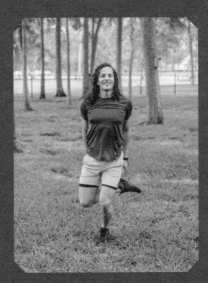 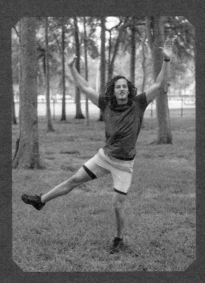

JUMPING JACK, ONE LEG: This is a dynamic warm-up for the upper and lower body. Position your body as for a standard jumping jack, but instead of jumping, keep one leg stationary as you touch your hands overhead with one leg pulsing out to the side.

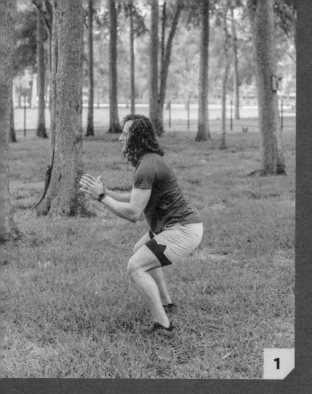

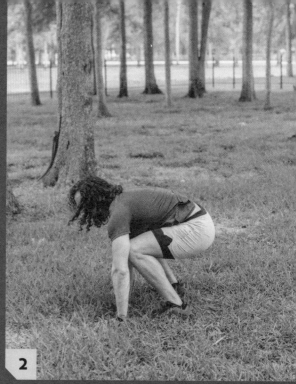

1 **2**

BURPEES: In a full squat, place the palms of your hands on the floor in front of your feet. Jump back into a push-up position, execute one push-up, return to the squat position, and jump up into the air while extending your arms overhead. This is a great total-body movement to build strength, explosiveness, and cardio fitness.

5 **6**

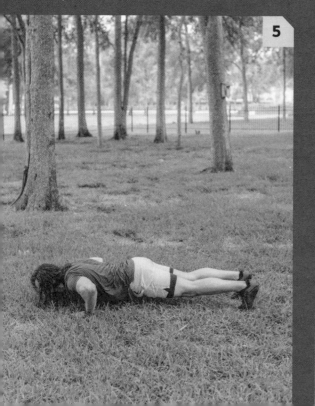

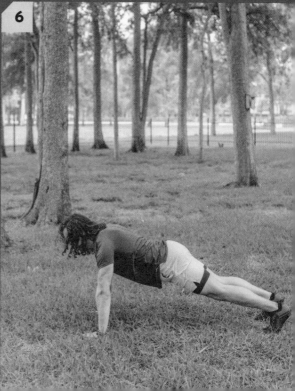

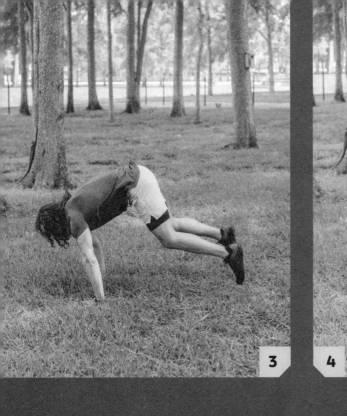

3

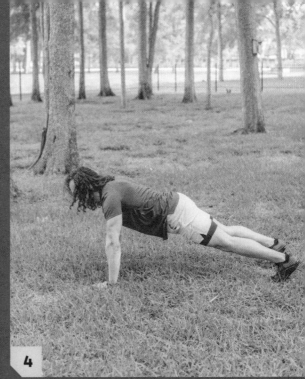

4

7

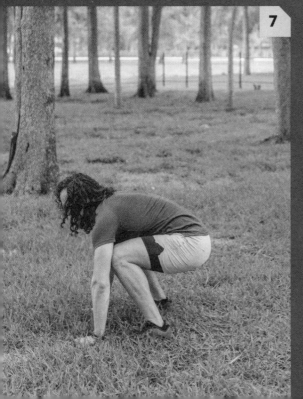

8

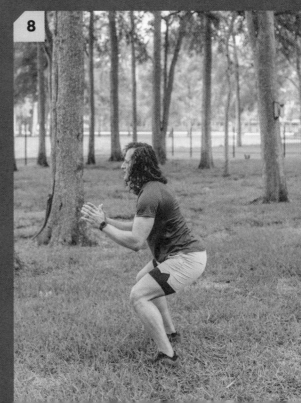

Prehab

I do a ton of rehab and even "prehab" exercises using TheraBands and the branded Flexbar for shoulder and wrist work. I've got a set of loop bands and long bands that go from "light" all the way to "very heavy," and I have an ever-growing library of mobility exercises that will increase the blood flow to previously injured areas or high-impact areas that regularly take a beating. My wrists, shoulders, knees, hips, and back all benefit significantly from regular use of my bands.

The term *bulletproofing* is popular for this type of training, and when you think of it in those terms, it's easy to make these exercises a priority in your weekly routine. The benefits are amazing in terms of preventing injuries.

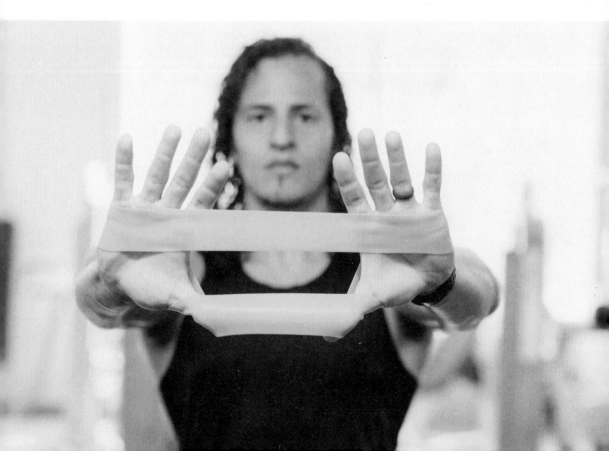

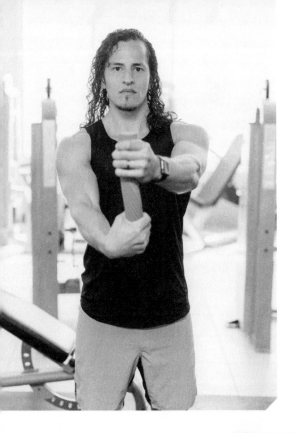
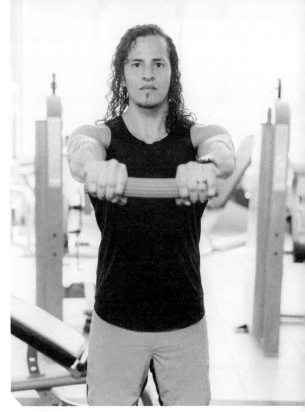
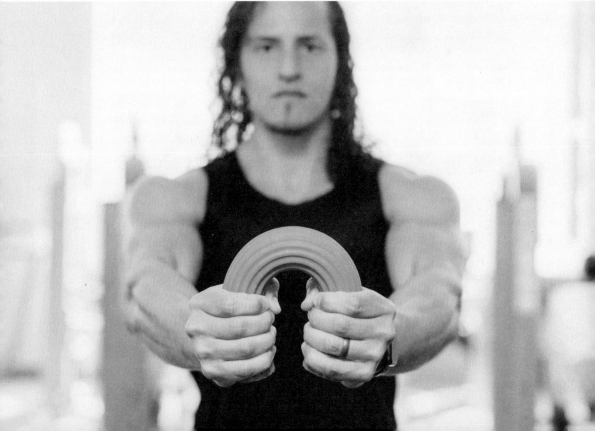

Shoulder Prehab Exercises

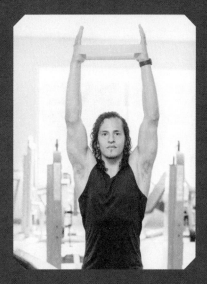
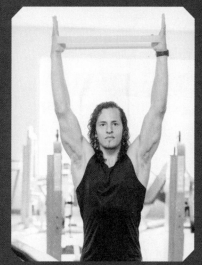

TOUCHDOWN: This exercise targets many of the muscles that stabilize your shoulders when they are in vulnerable positions above your head. Place your wrists inside a loop band and then extend your arms straight above, palms facing inward. Keeping your arms straight and focusing on using the muscles around your shoulder blades, push your arms away from each other, like you're a football referee making a "touchdown" signal. Return to the starting position and then repeat.

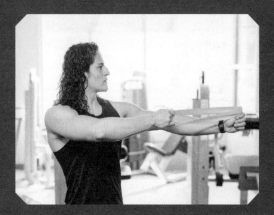
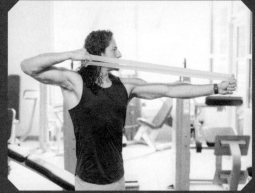

ARCHER PULLS, WITH BANDS: This is a single-arm exercise, but the non-working arm works to stabilize against the pull. It targets the middle back muscles, arms, and core. With your non-working arm, hold one end of a band (a long band for less tension, a loop band for more) straight out in front of your body. Like an archer, pull the other side of the band back toward your ear.

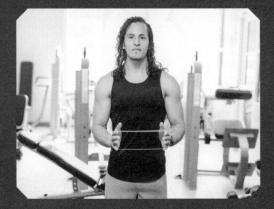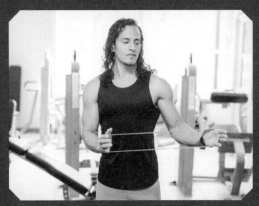

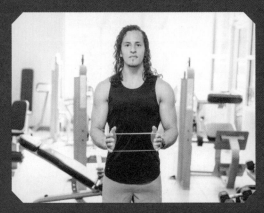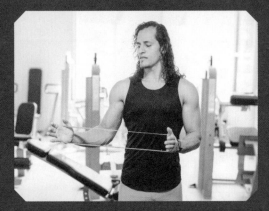

EXTERNAL ROTATION: Place a loop band around your wrists and then tuck your elbows to your side, making a 90 degree angle with your arms. Keeping your elbows at your sides, move your left hand away from your body by squeezing your shoulder blade in toward the middle of your back. Your right hand should remain stationary. Return to the starting position, under control. Then repeat on the opposite side.

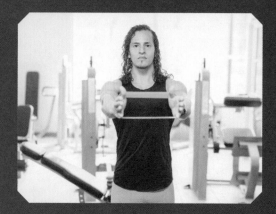

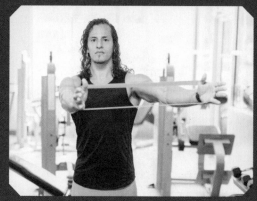

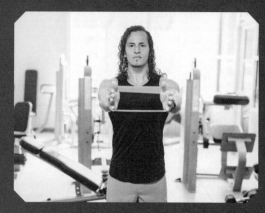

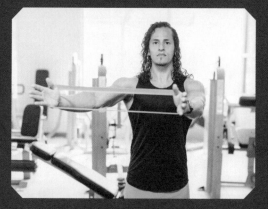

EXTENDED EXTERNAL ROTATION: This is like the external rotation exercise but with arms extended. With a loop band around your wrists, extend your arms straight out in front of you, palms facing inside. Move your left hand away from your body, squeezing your shoulder blade in. Under control, bring your hand back to its original position. Repeat on the other side.

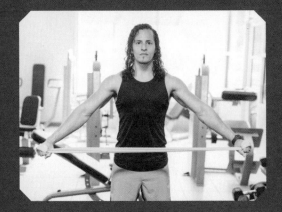 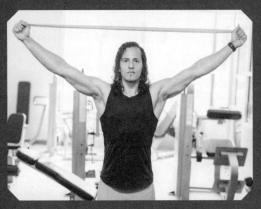

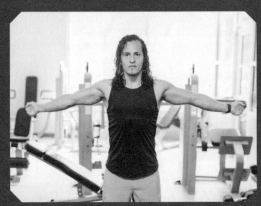 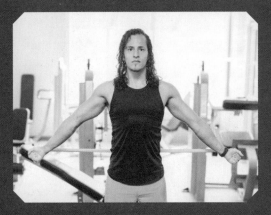

WIDE GRIP SWINGS: This exercise is all about increasing shoulder flexibility and stabilizing your shoulders from every imaginable angle. Grip a long band out wide, almost as wide as you can go while keeping the band near waist height. There should be a little bit of tension in the band. Keeping your arms straight, slowly raise both arms together until the band is above your head. Then, making sure not to overextend your shoulders, lower the band down behind your back. Once the band is back to waist height, raise it up behind you until it's above your head again, and then lower to your original starting position with your arms in front. Make sure to move your arms slowly and keep them straight throughout the exercise.

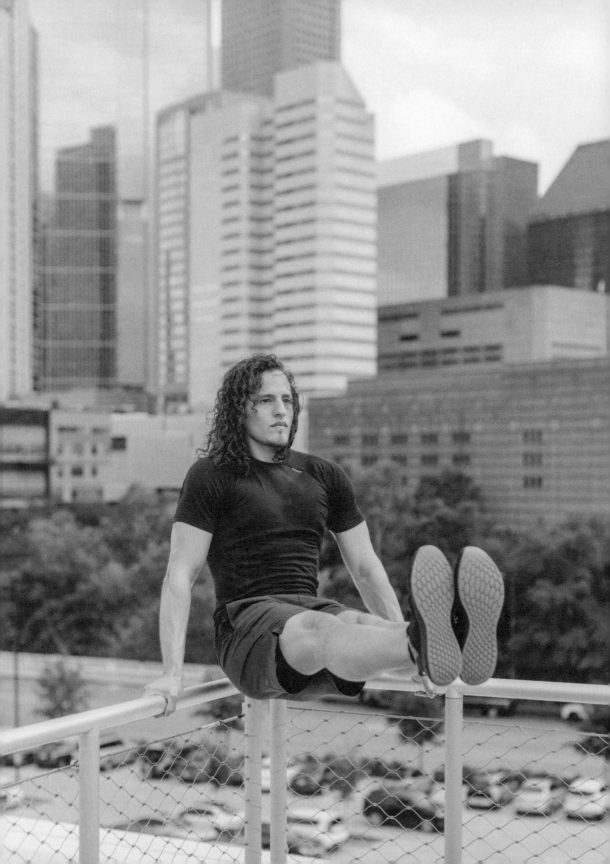

3

WORKOUTS

We can think of these workouts in tiers in the sense that there are a few movements people can do on their own without access to ninja gyms, and there are other more ninja-focused exercises that require special equipment. Our aim here is to promote general health, functional strength, and endurance. We can be good stewards of the bodies God gave us regardless of our starting point!

Now, this book isn't my exhaustive ninja training manual (perhaps that could be a future book someday). Instead, in this book I share some core things that you need to know and implement to achieve greater physical health and build functionality. These areas also directly impact ninja athletes (so they're still important!).

The first few weeks of a new fitness program are always the hardest. I say "few" because beginning a new training routine may be easy for some, and for others it may be a much greater shock to their system. Your body

 Always use discernment and check with your medical provider before beginning a new physical activity, especially something as high-intensity as ninja training.

may not be used to the new movements or specific types of exercise if you've never trained like that before! When I implement any new method of training, it always initially hits me the same way.

The first few weeks are also the most important because you're laying the foundation that everything else will be built upon. Your body *will* begin to adapt and become used to training. For the past fifteen years of my life, my workouts have never gotten easier to complete (mainly because I regularly increase the difficulty), but my body has become so accustomed to training that even though the workouts are tough, I'm not paralyzingly sore the next day. Instead, I'm ready for the next workout—of a different muscle group, of course. Training then becomes less about the physical torture and more focused on mental discipline and responsiveness to any form of difficulty that comes up in my life.

Body-Weight Interval Training

Here's the beautiful thing about body-weight exercises: no weights required! And usually, very minimal equipment—maybe just a pull-up bar or something similar that can hold your weight, like monkey bars at a park or even a door jamb.

Your body is the one thing you have to take with you wherever you go, so it makes sense that we should get better at moving it!

I'm obsessed with pull-ups. Assisted, weighted, one-arm, close grip, wide grip, lock-off . . . if you have access to a bar, the possibilities are endless for this simple, primal, all-purpose movement.

For a beginning pull-up routine, simply perform ten sets of standard chin-ups (palms toward you) to failure with 90 or 120 seconds of rest between each set, even if this means ten sets of one rep apiece. Track how many reps you are able to complete in each set. Perform this workout twice each week, and you'll see a difference!

Add ab straps to also get a great core workout. Even simply hanging on the bar for a couple minutes (if you can) will give you a killer grip workout. Start where you can and build a progressive routine.

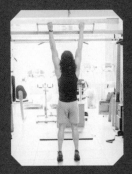 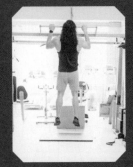

CHIN-UPS: The pull-up puts your hands in a pronated grip with your palms facing away from your body, while the chin-up uses a supinated grip with your palms facing toward your body. Each exercise emphasizes slightly different muscles, but both are great primary upper body resistance exercises to use regularly in your training. Hang from the bar using the forward hand grip and cross your lower legs. Bend your elbows to raise your body until your chin is at the level of the bar. Extend your elbows to return to the starting position.

WIDE GRIP PULL-UPS: This is like the normal pull-up, but more intense. With your palms forward and several inches beyond shoulder-width apart, grab the pull-up bar. Bend your elbows and pull yourself up until your collarbone is close to the bar. Slowly lower yourself to your starting position. Good luck.

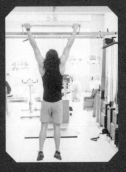 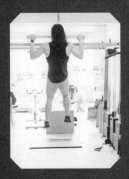

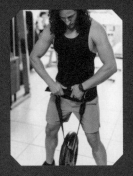 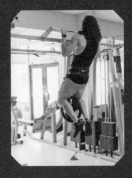

WEIGHTED PULL-UPS: These work lats, biceps, and forearms and are a great addition to any OCR athlete's grip-strength regimen. Use a weighted belt to add resistance to your pull-ups (palms forward) or chin-ups (palms inward). Be careful not to add more weight than you can handle. Also feel free to add resistance bands to help you with any type of pull-up training.

Push-Ups

There are many variations of push-ups. They are great for building upper-body strength and stabilizing your core (more on that next).

Here are a couple variations I utilize beyond the standard push-up. Do each exercise for 15 reps or for 30 seconds or to failure.

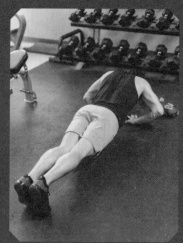

DIAMOND PUSH-UP: This is great for isolating your triceps and shoulders. In push-up position, place your hands close together on the ground, making a sort of diamond shape with your index fingers and thumbs. Lower yourself, push up, and repeat.

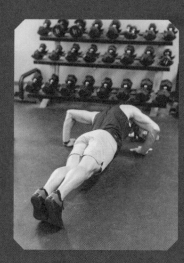

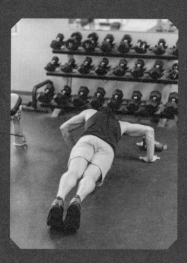

SINGLE ARM ISOLATION PUSH-UP: These are great for taking your push-up game to a whole new level, causing your arms to bear more weight than they would with a standard push-up. Place your hands on the ground slightly wider than shoulder width apart. In the upright plank position, slightly rotate your body to the right so that more of your weight is being supported by your left arm. Lower yourself, push up, and then repeat on the other side.

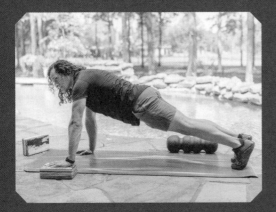
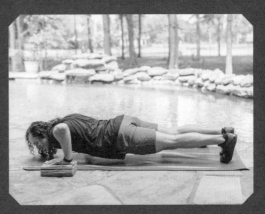

FOAM BLOCK PUSH-UP, ONE ARM DOWN: For a deeper push-up, use a foam block to elevate one hand higher than the other and perform push-ups in that position. Then do the same with the other side. Use both foam blocks simultaneously to get a deeper overall push-up variation.

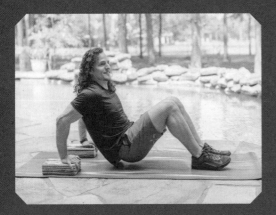
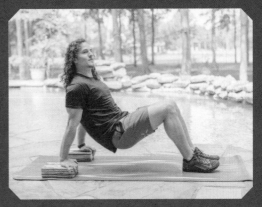

FOAM BLOCK DIPS: In a seated position on the floor, place foam blocks flat beneath your hands, extend your legs in front of you, bend your knees up, and keep your torso upright. Begin doing body-weight dips to strengthen your wrists and triceps. Flare your hands out if needed for extra wrist stability.

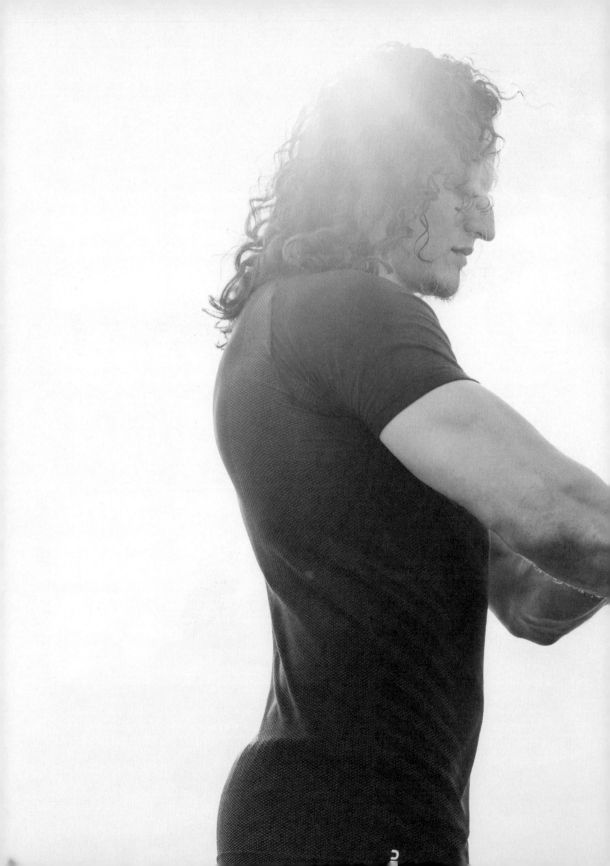

ANW SEASON 7: LAS VEGAS FINALS, STAGE 1, 2015, PART 1

Making it to the national finals my rookie year felt like a dream come true! Running stage 1 felt surreal. I had already run a few courses with great success and had been training hard to be prepared for the high-speed endurance courses that awaited me in Vegas.

As I ran across the Piston Steps, I remember thinking they were way wobblier and more unstable than I had anticipated. Thankfully, I had enough momentum off the starting runway to redirect my flailing body and still make it to the platform at the other end.

Then, I almost didn't make my jump up to the Propeller Bar obstacle. I hit the trampoline hard and with confidence, but the catch was so much higher up than I thought it would be. That's Vegas for you—everything is bigger and higher than in the qualifier and semifinal rounds! Once my hands grabbed the smooth surface of the propeller, I spun at least one full rotation before successfully grabbing the rope to the slanted landing platform.

The next obstacle was the Silk Slider and the cloth felt so thin and smooth in my hands that I had to grab a fistful of it and then double-wrap my wrists to better distribute the weight. I got as low as I could while stepping off the top and beginning my descent to the landing platform. As soon as I hit that inflatable pad, I sprawled out to stop my momentum because I had seen others land and continue forward off the other side of the platform into the water! I had also seen people let go too early and come up short, falling into the water and ending their season.

Once I got off the inflatable pad, I knew I could beat the rest of the course! But first I had to beat the ninja killer: the Jumping Spider. I had seen it take out so many ninjas over the years. It is an incredibly technical obstacle. You have to run *fast*, hit the trampoline in the *center*, stay *upright* as you fly forward through the air, and *simultaneously* open out your legs in order to land securely. So much to remember! Thankfully, I had it all locked in my muscle memory from months of training on that particular obstacle. I'm even more grateful for my years of dance, which gave me flexible hips and legs! Because of that foundation, I've never had issues with corridor body-propping obstacles. . . . *continued on page 82.*

Core

Your core is more than just your abs; it encompasses everything from your hips to your shoulders. Basically, it's all the muscles and joints that keep you upright and stable. Sounds pretty important, if you ask me! Too many people are so focused on getting six-pack abs that they neglect many other functions of their core. Without a strong core, an athlete is far more susceptible to injury and fatigue. All in all, if you have a stronger core, you will be a better, more capable athlete. Period. The exercises below are designed to strengthen all the areas of your core. But don't worry, your abs will feel it too.

I use a yoga mat (or a towel when I'm traveling) and do several minutes of isolated ab exercises focusing on endurance and power moves. Sometimes I'll go 7 to 10 minutes non-stop, switching exercises every 30 to 60 seconds. Other times I'll do 2 to 3 sets of about 3 minutes on with a 90-second rest, still switching exercises every 30 to 60 seconds. I do this type of ab routine 3 or 4 times each week.

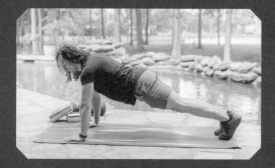

YOGA PLANK: This is like the "up" part of the push-up position. Get in this position and hold it.

CORE PLANK: Similar to a yoga plank, but resting on your elbows and toes. This centers most of your body weight on the core and is more challenging.

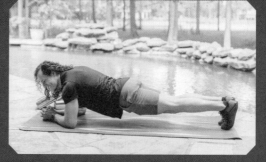

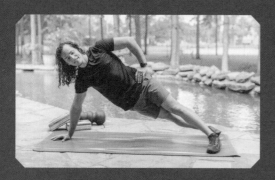

SIDE PLANK: This is a great way to activate and strengthen the core. Lie on your side with your knees bent, and prop your upper body up on your elbow. Raise your hips off the floor, and hold for 5 seconds. Rest for 10 seconds. Repeat 3 to 5 times on each side.

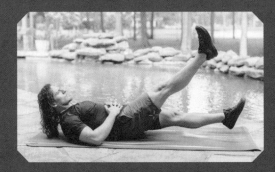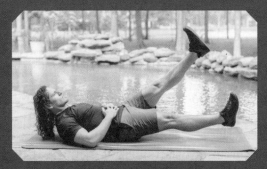

LEG LIFTS: Lie on your back with your hands on your stomach. Lift your heels, together, six inches off the ground, and hold. Then spread your heels apart and hold that position. Alternate legs.

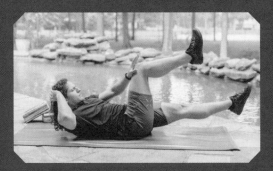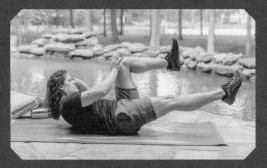

DEAD BUG: While lying on your back, lift both legs off the ground and straighten one leg while bending the other up toward your chest. Next, place the opposite hand against the bent knee and hold for 3 to 5 seconds before switching legs and hands. Repeat for a standalone ab workout or add other ab exercises.

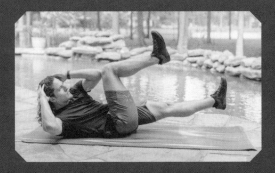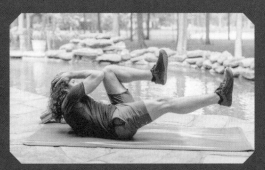

BICYCLE KICK: Lie face up and place your hands behind your head, supporting your neck with your fingers. Tuck your abs in and make sure the small of your back is pushed hard against the floor. Lift your knees in toward your chest while lifting your shoulder blades off the floor. Rotate to the right, bringing the left elbow toward the right knee as you extend the other leg into the air. Switch sides, bringing the right elbow toward the left knee. Alternate each side in a pedaling motion.

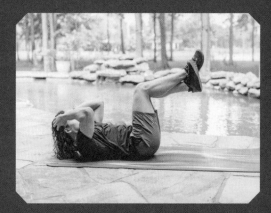 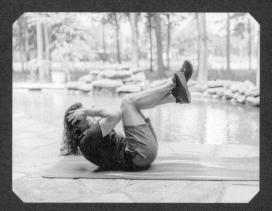

CRUNCHES: Lie down on the floor on your back and bend your knees, placing your hands behind your head or across your chest. Slowly contract your abdominals, bringing your shoulder blades about 1 or 2 inches off the floor. Exhale as you come up, keeping your neck straight and your chin up. Hold at the top for a few seconds and then slowly lower back down (but not all the way to a relaxed position). Repeat.

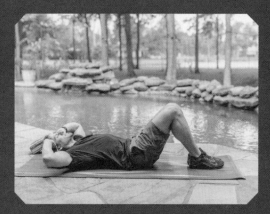 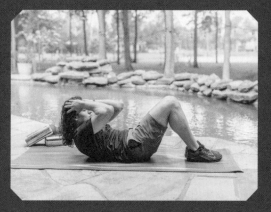

SIT-UP: Lie on your back on a mat with knees bent and feet flat on the floor. Cross your arms in front of your chest or place your hands at the sides of your head. Crunch your ab muscles to lift your shoulders off the mat. Hold for a second, then slowly come back down to starting position. Repeat.

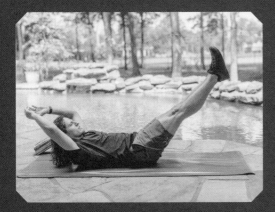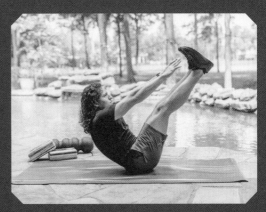

V-UP: Lie flat on your back with your arms above your head. Keeping your butt on the ground, lift both your torso and your legs so you form a *V* shape. Elevate your legs as high as you can, keeping them straight and together, and keep your back straight as you lift your torso up toward your thighs. Move your hands toward your feet as you lift into the *V*, hold, then lower to starting position, and repeat. Try to keep your movements slow and under control.

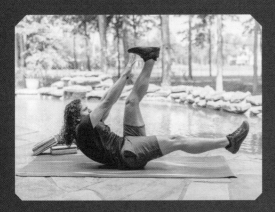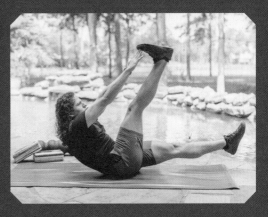

V-SIT, INDIVIDUAL LEGS: As above, but with one leg remaining on the ground. Repeat the exercise with the other leg.

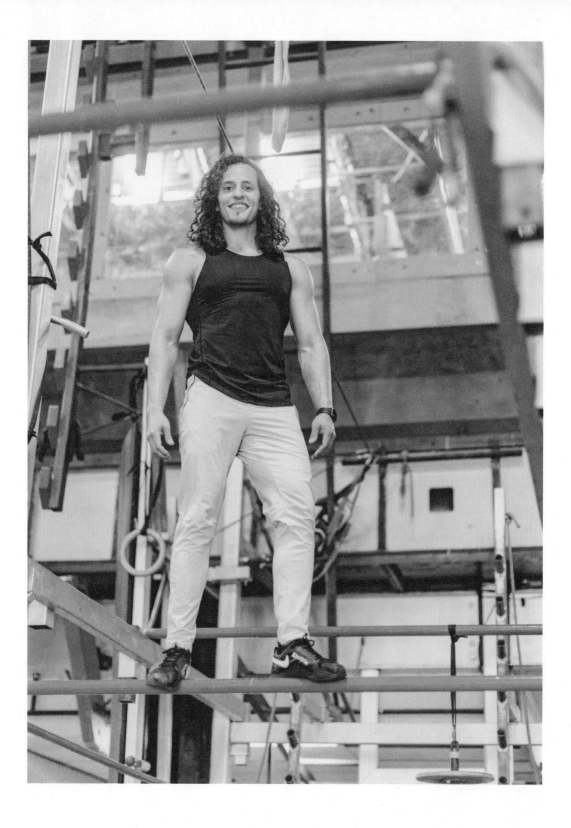

4

NINJA OCR TRAINING

Two-thirds of my weekly training is specialized athletic conditioning that directly translates to my sport of ninja OCR. I train in a way that also prepares me for competitions, the most important one being the show.

I do high-intensity dynamic obstacle training only a couple of times a week to avoid injuries (of which I have had many). The reasoning for this is twofold: (1) The training itself is dangerous (jumping, climbing, and potentially falling), and (2) the movements are so high-intensity that the muscles and tendons need time to recover. In the same way that a lifter or football player won't bench or squat two days in a row, an OCR athlete must hold to the principle of rest. Our bodies need time to recover.

THE ENDLESS ROPE

SOME OF MY favorite pieces of training equipment are a rowing machine, a treadmill, and my personal favorite, the endless rope. The rowing machine and endless rope engage most of the body and are great for cardiovascular endurance. You can aim to row for at least 30 minutes a day from 4 to 6 days a week, making sure to rest your muscles when needed.

The endless rope is great for the lats, biceps, upper back, and grip strength. This equipment is getting really popular among climbers. It's basically an upper-body treadmill because you can vary the speeds from as slow as a walking pace to as fast as an all-out sprint. You can even range it from almost zero resistance to extremely difficult to pull. It is a great cardio workout with a pretty simple concept—it simulates what it feels like to climb a rope but also has many other uses. I regularly use it for three or four different workouts.

The standard treadmill keeps me fit as a runner, which I need in ninja OCR. I love doing sprint intervals on it too. I have many different workouts that I do on each of these machines, from low intensity to high intensity.

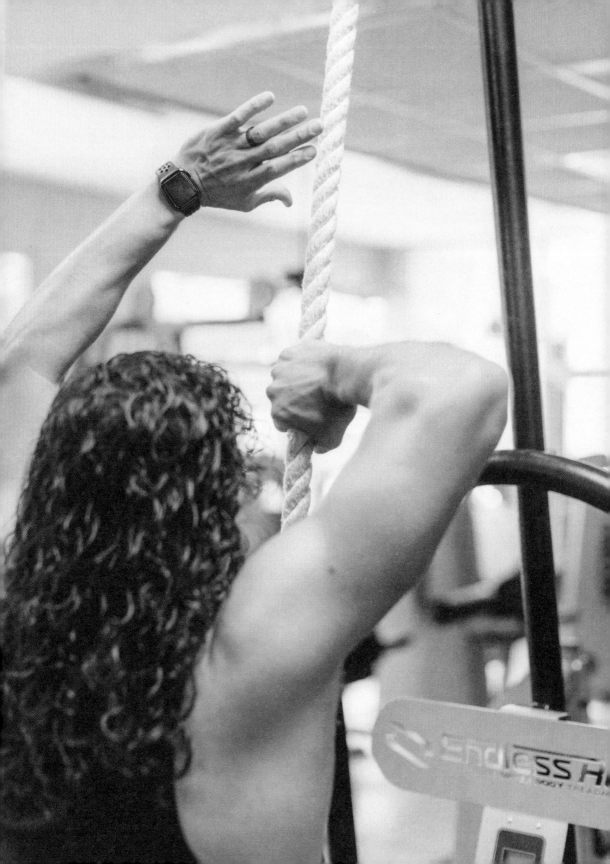

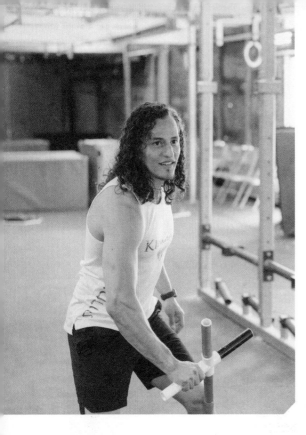
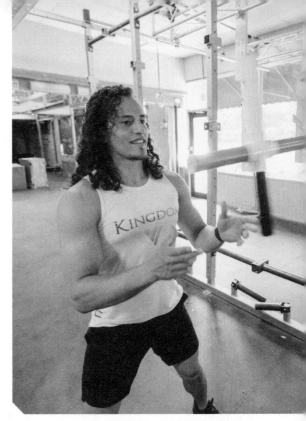
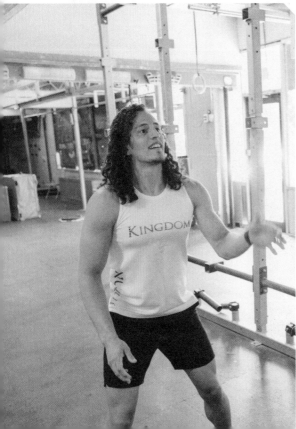
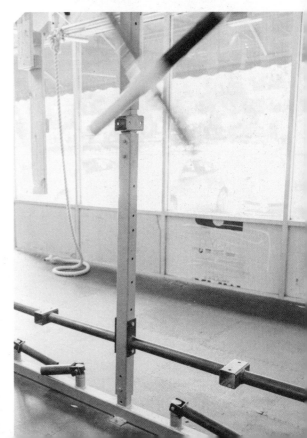

Coordination Drills

One thing I've learned over the years is just how beneficial coordination drills are, whether hand-eye, foot-eye, or a combination of the two. In an ever-evolving sport like ninja where you're constantly flying through the air and catching different types and sizes of holds, you *really* need to be aware of your surroundings and to be able to make split-second decisions with precise hand placement dialed in.

Some of my favorite drills are playing hacky sack (hands and feet), juggling, throwing and catching a small ball, or even getting creative and building something more elaborate. One of my personal favorite drills uses a small plus sign made out of PVC pipe. Each of the four ends is marked with a different color (duct tape works great!), and you toss it to your training partner and tell them which hand to use and which color pipe-end to grab.

There are many portable ways you can improve your hand-eye coordination by yourself, with a friend, or in groups. You can include these exercises as part of your warm-up routine, do them at the middle or end of your workouts, use them as a way to train on your rest days, and even take the tools with you to use as competition prep. They won't make you physically stronger, but the benefits translate well to almost every other sport and can even make or break you during the crux of your next competition. So find some coordination drills to add to your routine. These are just a few, so choose your favorites and stop missing those tricky catches!

The Quintuple Steps

This has been the first obstacle on *American Ninja Warrior* courses for many seasons. (It was *my* first-ever obstacle!) From the starting platform, you'll face five inclined steps spaced up to six feet apart. You have to jump from one to the next without falling into the water.

I remember it being WAY more intimidating than it looked on TV! I had envisioned myself easily bounding across the steps to immediately separate myself as a top-level athlete . . . but at the moment of truth, my legs felt like lead and wet noodles at the same time (if you can imagine that feeling). I ended up taking the more cautious three-step approach to the obstacle instead of one-stepping them. Like every challenge in life, the first step is always the hardest. Once I got through it I relaxed and, with renewed confidence, attacked the rest of the course with abandon and success!

The quintuple steps are all about lower body strength and agility. You'll need explosiveness in your quads, hamstrings, and calves. You'll also need knee and ankle flexibility. The key to conquering this obstacle is to just commit to it. Make sure your legs aren't floppy like noodles. Jump hard, push hard, and explode to the next step.

Hang Board

I think grip strength and confidence are the two most important attributes for any potential *Ninja Warrior* athlete. If you can't hold on to anything, you'll fall, especially at the end of a course when fatigue sets in.

CHALK LIFE

I love supporting my friends and the various brands of chalk companies that are out there. The funny thing, though, is that I rarely ever use chalk myself! I never train with it and use it only on certain occasions in competition.

Now, understand this: Every person is different—fearfully and wonderfully made. That goes for your body in general and your hands in particular, including the amount of chalk you personally might need. Your hands may often be dry as a bone, or you may suffer (at least suffer in the sport of ninja) by having hyperhidrosis, which makes your hands abnormally and excessively sweaty. You might be somewhere in between. You might have big hands; you might have small hands. You may prefer using powder chalk, or you might prefer liquid chalk. You might prefer your chalk in a sock ball in a bag for squeezing or in fine powder in a bucket for dunking.

Either way, understand what type of hands you're working with and then . . . well, then you learn to use the hands you've been dealt.

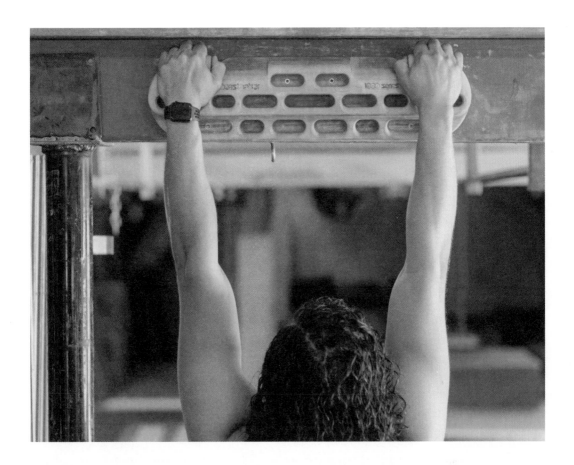

You might have big, strong muscles, but if you've got weak fingers, you'll reach your limit before you even get halfway through a course. A lot of times people will add rock climbing into their training regimen for improved grip and core strength. But if you're starting a new activity, tendons are at risk because it's all too easy to accidentally overtrain and injure a finger. Risk isn't worth it regarding finger tendons. Once damaged, they can take six to eight months to fully heal, sometimes longer! So listen to your body when it tells you to slow down. When a finger begins to ache, take a rest or stop what you're doing altogether, and train a different muscle group.

Using a rock-climbing hang board and a step, place your hands into one of the finger pockets and begin by just hanging. Once your fingers have gotten used to supporting your weight, you can slowly work in other body weight exercises with the hang board like pull-ups.

The Salmon Ladder

This is the supercool-looking obstacle made famous by the show *Arrow*. It's a tough obstacle for beginners but a must-have for those who want to compete on the show someday. On this intimidating obstacle, you hang on a bar that rests in rungs and then use your whole body to jump the bar to a higher set of rungs. It requires upper-body strength, coordination, timing, and explosiveness.

To conquer the Salmon Ladder, you need to practice explosive pull-ups. If you can do a clapping pull-up, then you can do the salmon ladder.

The secret is to learn how to hold the bar. Make sure to grab the bar at shoulder width. Hands too close and you won't have control of the bar. Hands too wide and you might pinch a finger. Grab the bar with both hands in the forward grip (pull-up style), or use a mixed grip, with one hand facing toward you and the other facing away from you. Forward grip is fine to use, but when you're tired, the bar will spin out of your hands. So I don't recommend using it if the Salmon Ladder is a later obstacle in a course. I have always used mixed grip because the bar does not spin when you hold it like that. Just keep in mind that one hand will likely go higher due to the mixed grip, and it takes practice to keep both hands level.

While hanging on the bar, engage your core muscles, pull up slightly on the arms to 45 degrees, and then drive your knees to your chest. During that weightless moment at the apex of the explosive movement, pull the bar out, up, and into the next rung. Remember to absorb the impact because it's an aggressive obstacle, and if you relax too much you won't be able to hold on. Find the perfect balance of holding on tightly but not over-gripping or pumping out your forearms too soon.

Stay focused and practice each style to be able to use this movement whenever necessary.

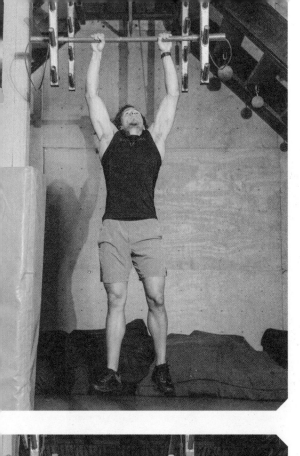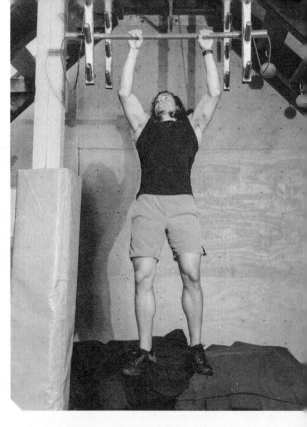

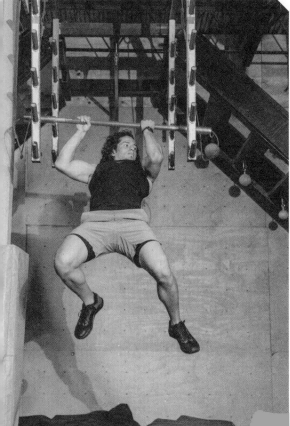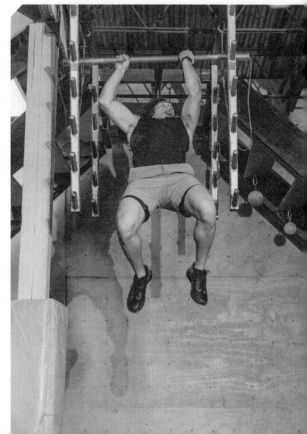

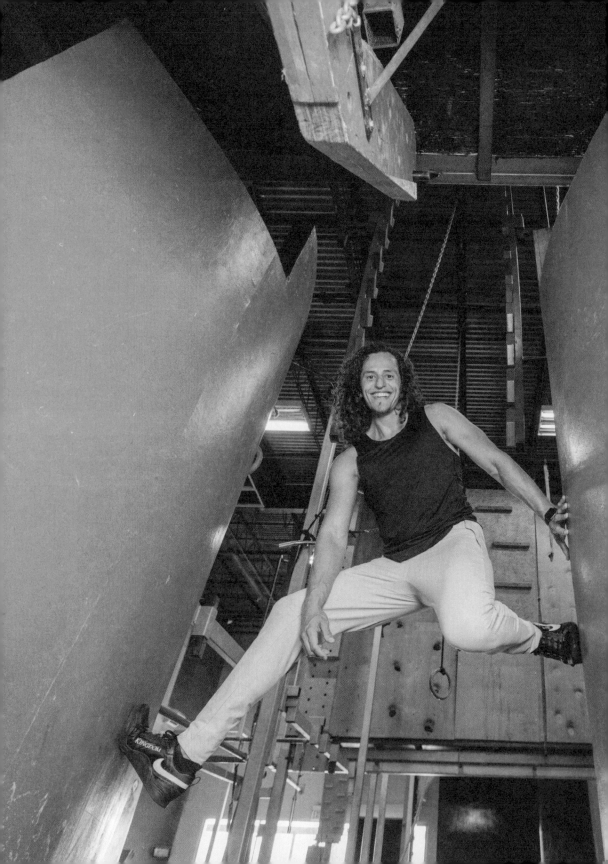

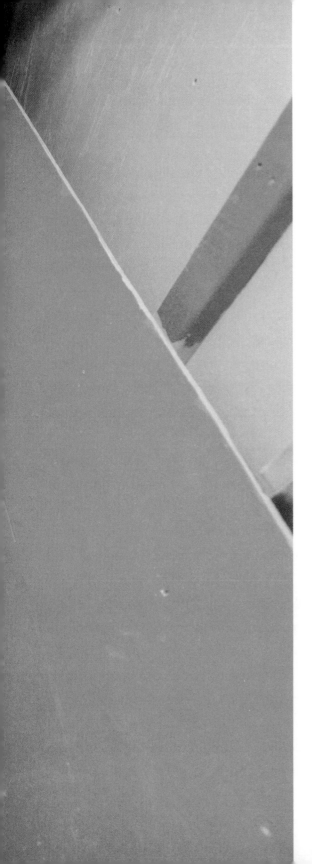

The Jumping Spider

STEP ONE: Learn how to jump off a trampoline. Practice jumping forward for distance and also up for height. For the Jumping Spider, you have to jump high and also far in order to stick the landing easily.

STEP TWO: Work on lower body flexibility in the hamstrings, hip flexors, and ankles because this obstacle is very dynamic and abrupt with the landing.

STEP THREE: Warm up well, make sure you have proper landing pads in place (if necessary), and then begin attempting the obstacle. While airborne, don't lean too far forward or backward. You want to land perfectly upright between the walls. Shoes also play a huge role in this obstacle because rubber soles will stick much better than just foam.

Once you master the landing, you can try shortening the runway, pulling the trampoline farther from the walls incrementally, or even dropping from a higher block down onto the trampoline to start.

The Warped Wall

This is the mega obstacle—the one that has conquered many aspiring ninjas. It's also one of the most dangerous obstacles. One wrong step and you could have a broken leg.

And then there's the Mega Wall: an eighteen-foot warped wall that *ANW* competitors can choose to attempt at the end of the qualifiers course . . . if they make it that far. It is a great incentive to go big or go home because you can win $10,000 by completing it. But you run the risk of missing and having to go to the fourteen-foot wall and finishing the course with a much slower time. The Mega Wall is such an intimidating obstacle! But once I heard it was being introduced in competition, I trained my butt off (literally) and was ready to conquer it two years in a row.

When first attempting a warped wall, never start out at maximum output. (Also, the older you are the more you should warm up prior to attempting it.) Begin at 60 to 70 percent of your max output and focus on form and technique.

You need a fast approach. Then, once you are on the wall, accelerate up it, keeping your chest high. On your last step, add a forward jump for increased height, and reach.

Once your technique looks and feels good, begin to increase your speed and effort little by little. After you've grown comfortable on the wall and built up your confidence, begin increasing your output to eventually use your maximum strength and attempt higher walls. Though warped walls may vary by gym (based on angle, traction, and length), the technique remains the same.

Additionally, for increased traction, make sure to wipe your shoes with a damp towel or use your hands to rub away dust and dirt and heat up the rubber.

Only after your technique is good should you begin gradually increasing your speed and power up to 100 percent—and that's just for the regular

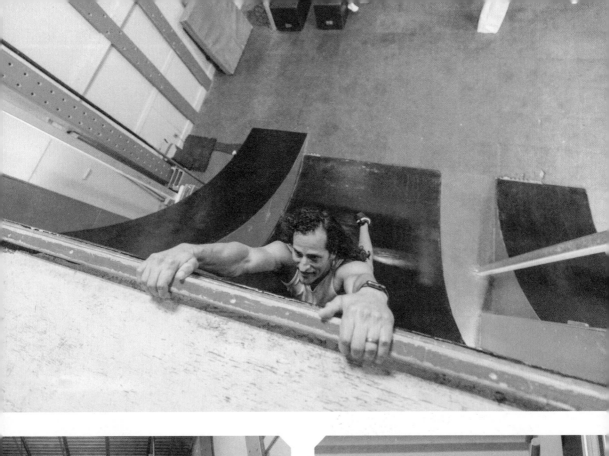

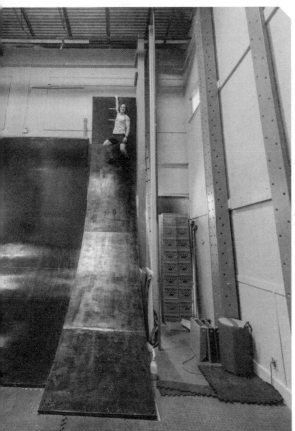

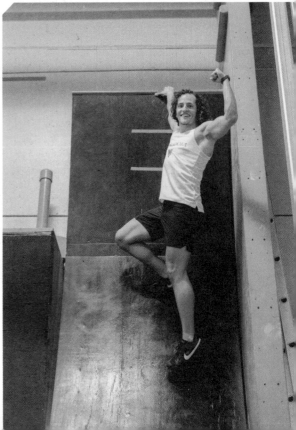

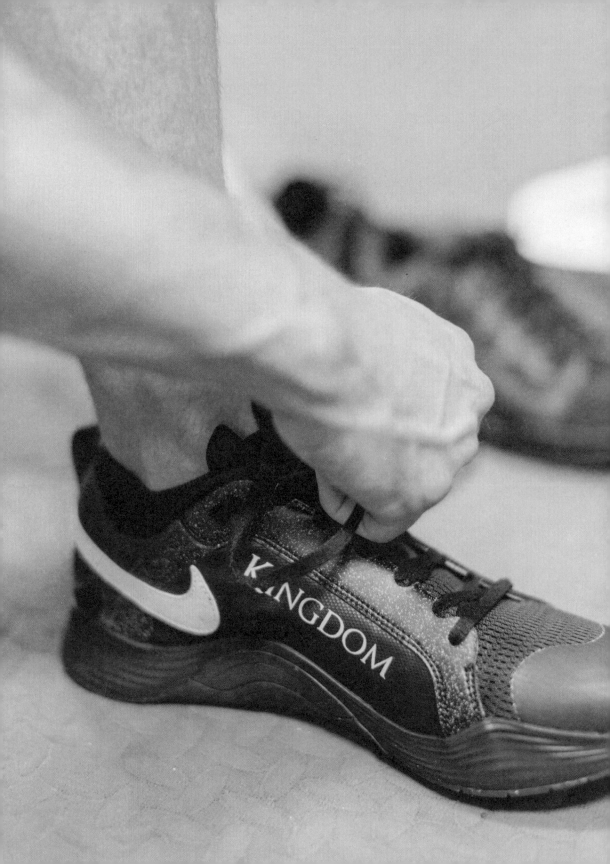

SHOES MAKETH THE NINJA

UNLIKE MOST SPORTS, there are not a lot of shoes built specifically for the needs of ninja athletes. Running and parkour shoes have filled the gap for years and years, but I believe there is coming a day when there will be a wealth of specialized shoes for this new and growing sport.

Honestly, you can start out with any shoe that has a good, smooth rubber sole. I often tell my students and friends that you want something that feels good on your foot, gives you support where you need it, has rubber on the bottom instead of simply foam, and has a lot of flat surface area on the sole to maximize your traction on the course.

Keep in mind that the shoe has to maintain traction on plexiglass, wood, and metal surfaces, sometimes gripping vertically, horizontally, laterally, or diagonally. Shoes can easily make or break you on a course, especially with money like the $10,000 Mega Wall at stake. Whatever your shoe, just please remember to wipe the dust or chalk off your soles before attempting any kind of Spider Wall obstacle!

wall. The only way you're ever going to make it up a massive Mega Wall is to go 100 percent, but you must already have great wall technique and already know how to fall properly if you're going to play with that beast of an obstacle. Good luck!

How to Fall Safely

The number one thing you should learn quickly as a ninja athlete is how to fall correctly. While training or competing, falling is a regular part of the sport.

You must never lock your joints when falling. Don't lock your wrist, elbows, knees or ankles. Keep things bent and fluid as much as you can.

Always try to absorb the impact by continuing the motion instead of stopping yourself instantly. If you are falling toward your feet, bend your knees and even squat into the landing before rolling away, if you can. That will keep the force from hitting your body all at once.

If you fall toward your upper body, begin to catch yourself with your hands but allow yourself to fall into the mat and try to roll through the fall if you can. Again, you want to disperse the force as much as possible from any single point on your body.

If you fall backward from a lache, do not put your hands down behind you to try to catch your fall. Instead, bring your arms in toward your body and trust your training and the mat beneath you. Better to have the air knocked out of you than to break an arm.

The best thing you can do as a ninja athlete is practice "trust falls" onto mats from varying heights, and practice bar laches and landing on your back into a thick cushion. Falling happens, but the more you have experienced it in a controlled environment, the less damaging it can be in the heat of the moment.

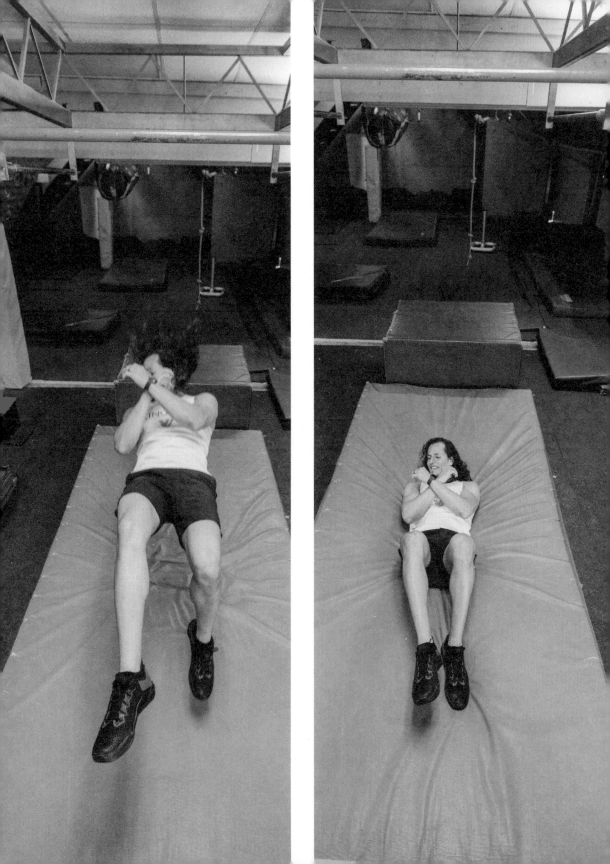

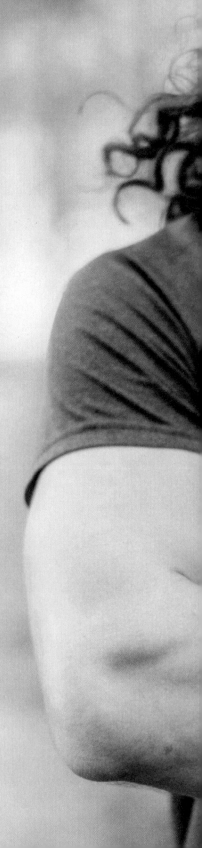

ANW SEASON 7: LAS VEGAS FINALS, STAGE 1, 2015, PART 2

Continued from page 59...

Once I was through the Spider, I ran across the Sonic Curve and swung to the small landing platform. Wall runs aren't that tough, but when you have to jump away from the wall and change your direction, then grab a rope in midair, swing, and land precisely on a log platform . . . that's where it can get difficult! Some competitors took many swings before landing, and others couldn't get both hands on the rope and slid into the water. Some even landed but couldn't maintain their balance and fell. I was very happy to make it through.

Next on the lineup was the Warped Wall, which was a lot harder than the ones in qualifiers and semis. The runway for this wall was shorter, and you dropped into it like a skate park half pipe. That kind of start throws you off balance and forces you to be more explosive in order to reach the top. In addition, by that point you're tired, and you've been sucking in dusty air the last minute and a half while sprinting through the front half of the course. Honestly, I didn't think I had made the grab because of how different it was from the normal wall, but then my fingers grasped the top lip of the wall, and I locked on as tightly as I could! Two obstacles left!

The Coin Toss obstacle was literally a toss-up because anything can happen with tricky, dynamic agility obstacles. You run fast and light-footed and pray that you don't step too far on the front or back end. If you do, the coins will flip, and you fall. I ran on a prayer and was able to make it safely across.

The Triple Swing is a bar lache obstacle. Easy to do in training, but stressful and difficult when you're racing against the last seconds of the clock and you are out of gas. I knew what needed to be done and that I could complete it, so I took as deep a breath as I could and finished that course. I'll never forget the feeling of hitting that stage 1 buzzer and then immediately feeling like my throat was on fire and I was going to pass out!

Then straight to the interviews I went!

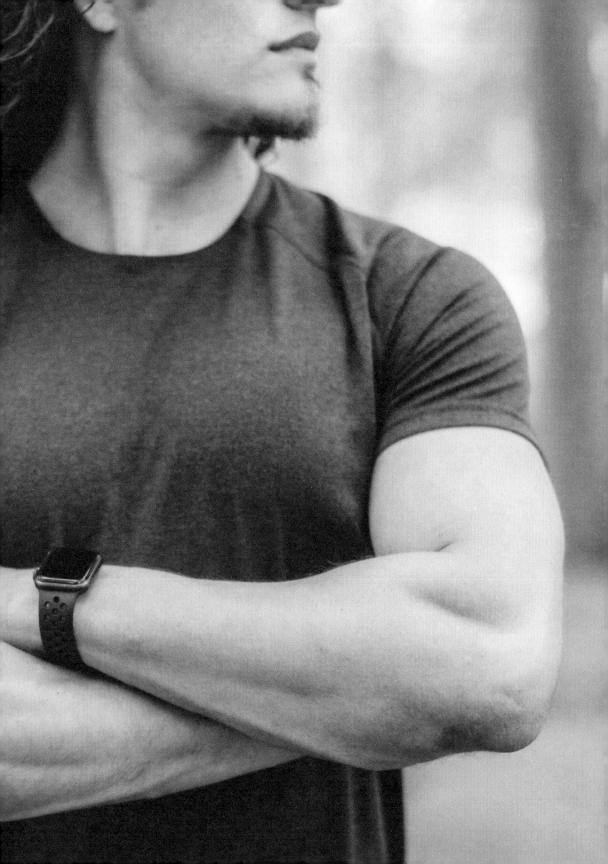

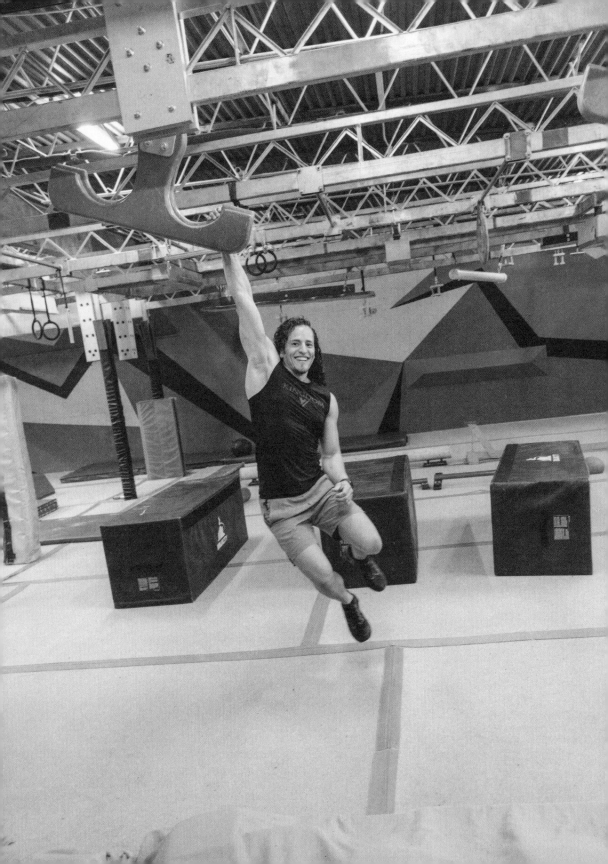

Building a Home Ninja Gym

It's really cool to see ninja competitions in other countries. I love the way cultural differences show in their courses.

One time Abby and I were in Nice, France—a big touristy spot on the French Riviera—supporting a good friend, Mathis Owhadi, who is a dual citizen. He was competing for *Ninja Warrior France* and didn't want to go on the adventure alone. We had a great time cheering him on. Their format is very different from *American Ninja Warrior*, which is really interesting. For *American Ninja Warrior* we have the qualifiers, then the semis, then the national finals, where if you hit a buzzer you move on and if not you're out of the competition. In France, half of the course is split into a fork—after the first four obstacles you choose between course A and course B. They have a Mega Wall similar to what we have in America—but if you conquer the wall in the qualifiers, you get to skip it until the finals.

You don't need to travel the world or move to a city with a ninja gym to train. In the world of ninja, the home gym is probably one of the main ways newcomers train. There are more than a dozen companies that specialize in custom backyard or home rig setups. There are companies that build resources or obstacles and sell them to gyms or individuals.

Obviously the most expensive way to do an at-home course is to have it professionally built. But as with many other things in life, you usually get what you pay for. Of course, doing it on your own requires a lot more time, energy, effort, and sweat. And then there's kind of a hybrid way to engage a builder to bring your vision to life. I've seen at-home builds run cheap, and I've seen them run very expensive when dropping posts deep into the ground and installing gymnastics-grade cushioning to guard against falls.

The vast majority of backyard courses are for children, to supplement their training at gyms. If you're a competitive athlete, there's nothing better than access to a gym where you can do a 30-foot rope climb and run courses that are ever-changing. Once you build a backyard course, you can keep adding to it and occasionally changing things up. Some people love that. Others don't.

You can find schematics online, purchase the designs, and then purchase things at Home Depot to add to your own course. If you're a carpenter or are handy in any way, you can just type in "backyard ninja course" and find all kinds of ideas. It all depends on what you want, what you can afford, and what fits best with your personality and goals for the course.

At my house, I have a traditional home gym setup, with supplementary training equipment to help me build strength for when I head to the ninja gym to run courses.

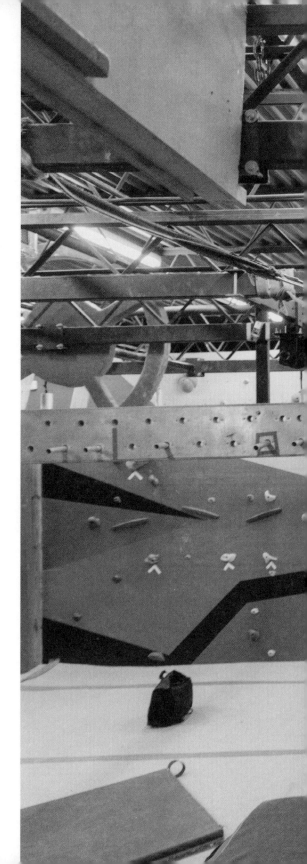

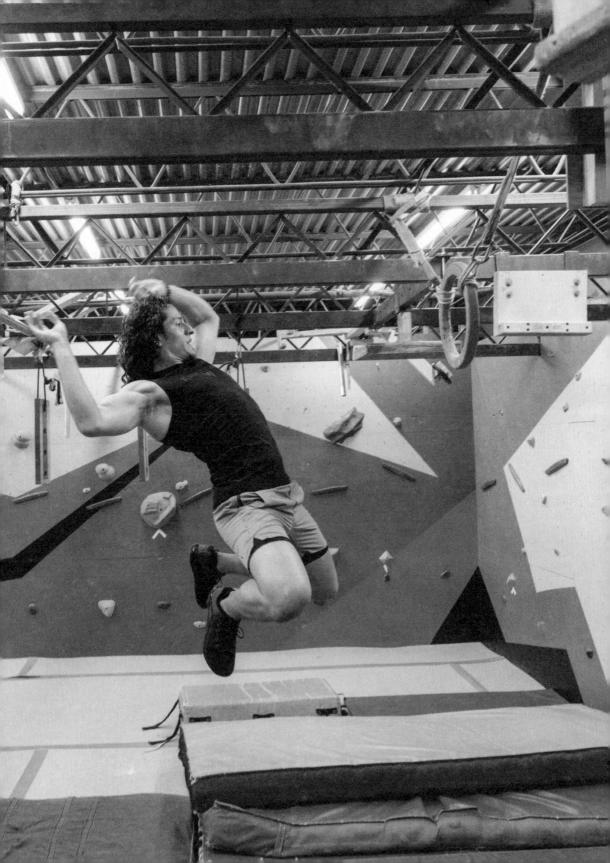

My top things every home ninja gym should have

Whatever route you take for a home gym, here are five things I think should be in every home course.

QUINTUPLE STEPS: These are easy to make and tough to defeat. There are many versions and variations of this ninja staple—short, long, high, and low.

SALMON LADDER: Make sure the supports for the rungs are secure and can support your weight.

CLIFFHANGER: On this tough obstacle, contestants must swing from one wall to the next and climb hand-over-hand using individual wooden rails. Contestants must use a side-to-side swing and a forward-and-backward swing to complete the Cliffhanger. This engages the whole body and is great for grip strength. Make sure you have different-size ledges based on age and ability: 2-inch banister, 2-inch flat beveled ledge, and 1.5-inch flat beveled ledge.

ADJUSTABLE BAR LACHE LANE: Simply put, ninja athletes need to be able to lache (swing from one hanging bar to another), and an adjustable home set will allow an athlete to vary the elevation and distance between bars. You can upgrade to a multilevel setup for advanced training.

STRAPS AND HANGING HOLDS: You can hang cannon balls, nunchucks, rings, trapeze bars—anything you can find to increase your grip strength and challenge yourself!

ROCK CLIMBING HOLDS: Whether on a climbing wall, connected to your cliffhanger, or added on posts to help climb up to an obstacle, rock climbing holds are a great addition to any course.

CRASH PADS: Crash Pads are vitally important to have beneath any laches or obstacles that are high enough that if you fell you could be injured. These are abundantly available online in various thicknesses and are usually made of foam, but there are some inflatable versions as well. I've even seen layers of tire rubber make for a decent cushion.

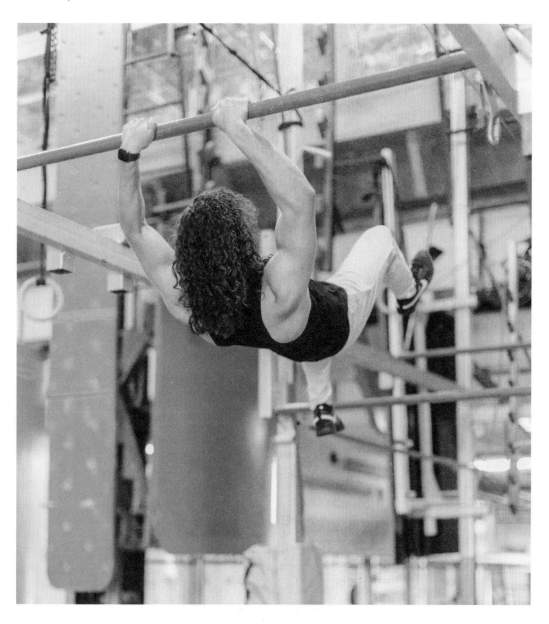

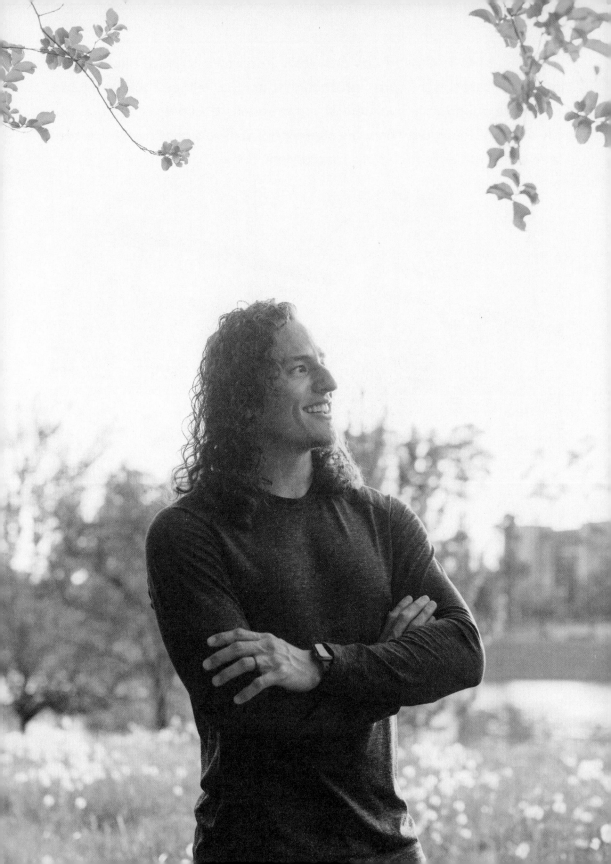

5

RECOVERY

How you rest and recover is just as important as how you train. If you're not smart about recovery, you can increase your risk of injury and possibly lose any gains you made in your workouts.

Over the years I have encountered and befriended many physical therapists, chiropractors, and Airrosti specialists who've spent their lives working on the body. Being able to ask their advice and receive their care has been hugely beneficial for me.

Let's Roll

I use a foam roller on a regular basis and keep one close by at all times. Sometimes I use a foam roller during my warm-up routine to roll out an area that needs extra attention, such as my calves, IT bands, or lats. Other times I use a roller during my workouts between sets in order to loosen up muscles I just pushed to their limits.

I almost always use one after my workouts to relax my aching, sore muscles and loosen up any knots that may have formed during my training. I keep a roller at the gym, one at my home, and a portable one in my travel bag at all times. It's an invaluable piece of workout gear that any athlete should learn how to use. I love finding new methods, techniques, or workouts to use with my foam rollers.

The Rollga foam roller is my go-to foam roller that I highly recommend to athletes because of its ergonomic design. (Important to note here—I recommend some brands below, but I am not sponsored by any of them and have not received anything for their mentions. These are just brands I personally use and enjoy!) Foam rolling can relieve muscle tenderness and soreness in the days after workouts when the muscles are fatigued. Foam rolling and other SMR rolling devices help to move fluid through your fascia and connective tissue layers, keeping those tissues hydrated, which is important for proper tissue repair. Here are a few sample movements for big muscle groups:

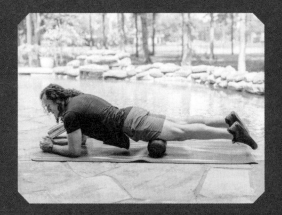

QUADRICEPS ROLL: Kneel on the floor and place the foam roller right in front of both knees. From there, bring your body forward to the floor, and ensure that your hips and body are grounded to prevent any form of back pain. Once the roller is under your quads and your body is on the floor, begin rolling forward and backward to massage the femoris.

HAMSTRING ROLL: From a seated position on the floor, feet forward, place a foam roller underneath your leg and gently push your body back and forth, engaging the roller from glute to knee. After 30 seconds to a minute of rolling, switch legs.

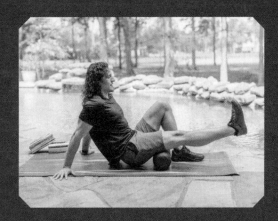

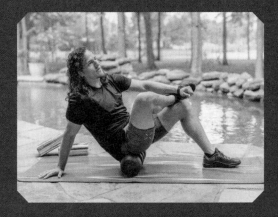

HIP ROLL FIGURE FOUR: For most people, sitting all day at work really contributes to hip tightness. Sit on the roller and reach your right arm back, planting your right hand on the floor a few inches behind you. Cross your right ankle over your left knee in a figure four position. Shift your weight to the right hip/glute area and roll back and forth a few inches in each direction for about 30 seconds. Repeat on the opposite side.

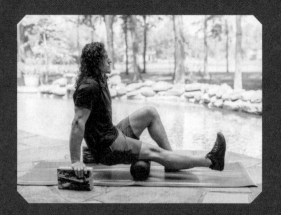

HAMSTRING ROLL, FOAM BLOCK: Position one hamstring on top of the foam roller while the opposite foot is flat on the ground with your knee up for stability. Hold foam blocks to elevate your torso. Set your hamstring and body weight down onto the roller and begin rolling back and forth as long as desired. Do the same with the other leg.

SHOULDER ROLL: Position yourself on your knees with the foam roller in front of you. Lean forward, and with straight arms and hands on top of the roller, push it back and forth, gently applying pressure onto your shoulders. Do as long as desired.

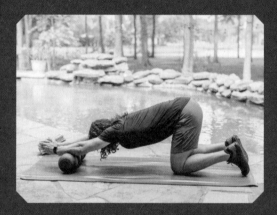

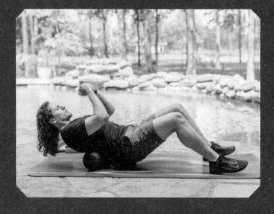

BACK ROLL: Lay your back down onto the roller and begin rolling back and forth as desired.

Apart from my warm-up, I also stretch a few times each week, usually while watching a show with Abby or listening to a podcast. For both upper body and lower body, I have a list of my problem areas to target and my favorite stretches that I hit each time. Since I was a dancer for a number of years, I have a high bar of where I want my flexibility to be, and I work hard to maintain it. Usually I begin with a dynamic movement (or pulse) through the stretch for around 30 seconds before fully sitting into and holding the stretch for up to two minutes before switching sides and then changing stretches. Stretching may seem tedious and often painful, but it is well worth it in the eyes of any dedicated, disciplined athlete.

I'll end each workout with dynamic stretches, mobility movements, and static stretches. Static stretching requires you to move a muscle as far as it can go without feeling any pain, then hold that position for 20 to 45 seconds. Here are a few static stretches I really value:

FOAM BLOCK LUNGE STRETCH: While in a deep lunge, hold foam blocks for stabilization and with every exhale sink a little bit deeper. Repeat with the other leg.

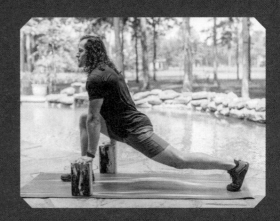

SHOULDER STRETCH: Stand tall, feet slightly wider than shoulder-width apart, knees slightly bent. Place your right arm across the front of your chest, parallel to the ground. Bend the left arm up and use the left forearm to ease the right arm closer to your chest. You will feel the stretch in the shoulder. Repeat with the alternate arm.

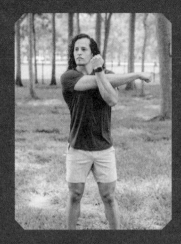

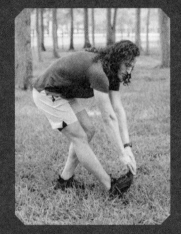

HAMSTRING STRETCH: Standing with your legs shoulder-width apart, step forward with your right foot. Keeping the front leg straight, slowly bend your back leg as you reach for your front foot. You will feel the stretch in the hamstring of the right leg. Repeat with the other leg.

QUAD STRETCH: Standing with your legs shoulder-width apart, bend one leg behind you and pull your foot up toward your glute. Use one or both of your hands to keep the foot there. This will stretch out the muscles in your quadriceps. Repeat with the other leg.

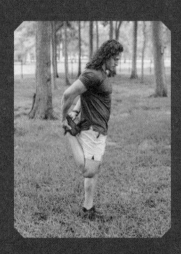

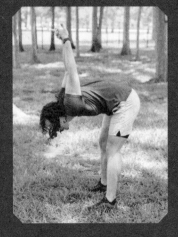

BACK STRETCH: Stand with your feet about shoulder-width apart and hold your arms behind you, interlocking your fingers with palms facing away from you. With your knees slightly bent and your back straight, slowly bend forward at your hip. At the same time, extend your arms away from your body as far as possible. You'll feel this stretch at your shoulders, your lower back, glutes, and hamstrings.

Massage, Ice, Compression

I own several Theragun massage guns and use them quite often in tandem with my warm-up, cool down, and recovery routines. These used to be within the distinct purview of professional team athletes, limited to training rooms, but they're now available to the general public, and I highly recommend them!

I own HyperIce Normatec Compression sleeves for arms, legs, and hips and use them regularly for recovery and inflammation management.

I use a hot tub and cold plunge routine on a weekly basis and strongly encourage every competitive athlete who has access to these tools to do the same for muscle and joint recovery. Even if you don't, you can do as I do and end every morning shower with a change from hot water to a minute or two of freezing cold water. I especially love to do this when I am traveling and need to wake up for an event or competition. The rapid shift from hot to cold water will close up the pores, wake up the nervous system, and remind you that you are not only alive but also disciplined to chase after your goals and dreams. It's a great way to begin each day.

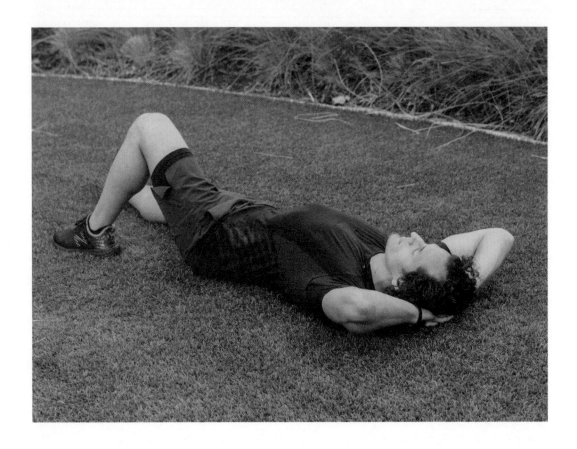

Rest Days

One of the greatest things I have learned over my years as an athlete is to listen to my body. When it comes to rest and recovery days, I certainly have them scheduled weekly, but I also occasionally have impromptu rest days that weren't planned. Some days I wake up and my body says, "Go for it!" Other days I wake up and my body says, "Let's take it easy today. Please go easy on me."

Scheduled or not, the best thing you can learn to do is listen when your body speaks and adjust accordingly. Injuries happen when I push myself too hard on days my body is asking for rest.

On my scheduled rest days I still try to do some sort of movement-based activity, like go for a walk, catch some rays by the pool and swim, take a light jog, stretch and do rehab exercises at home, or do a fun activity with friends or family.

On my days that I'm scheduled to train but just not feeling it, I tone down my workouts from something like 80 to 100 percent effort to more like 50 to 70 percent of my maximum level of effort, exertion, and impact.

As an additional tool, if you're serious about being on top of your recovery, there are a number of fitness recovery tracking devices that monitor your heart rate variability while you sleep and give you a wellness score each morning to help you determine your level of "readiness" for the day. I use one regularly, and it helps put words to how my body feels when I wake up each day.

However you choose to do it, make sure that your body gets the adequate rest it needs to fully recover. Otherwise, you won't benefit as much from your next workout, or worse, you could get injured if you are not careful.

Sleep

Sleep is *huge* for me! Sleep is key for both muscle recovery and mental health. My wife, Abby, and I don't have kids yet, so it is easy for us to make sleep a massive priority. (Even after we have kids we'll prioritize sleep, but I know it will be a lot different and more difficult. It'll be a different season of life, and we'll cross that bridge when we get to it.)

If you're wondering why you're not recovering well or making your desired gains, it could be due to lack of proper sleep. The number of hours each person needs varies by age, lifestyle, and many other factors. There is no perfect formula, but as an athlete I try to regularly get seven to nine hours of sleep a night. If I ever don't get enough sleep during the night, I try to take a power nap (again, a healthy nap duration varies for everybody—there is no "one size fits all" mold).

Abby often makes fun of me because I can literally let myself sleep anywhere at any time. I've slept on planes, on trains, in cars, at concerts, at competitions, and even at church once or twice! When my body gets tired and I choose to let it, I will sleep. I recognize that I am blessed in this regard, and I might as well take advantage of it!

Grounded

Ever hear someone say that they enjoy long walks on the beach? Well, that's me! Seriously, I absolutely love walking barefoot anywhere outside. The feeling of grass, dirt, or sand beneath my feet . . . there's just nothing else quite like it.

Additionally, there is a lot of research out there about "grounding" with the earth. The earth gives off an electromagnetic field that can help improve sleep, reduce inflammation, enhance blood flow, and increase HRV (heart rate variability), not to mention the variety of benefits of increased sun exposure and many other perks. I encourage you to check it out on your own if you are interested. All I know is that ever since I was a child, I have loved to unwind and relax by going for a barefoot walk outside.

Twenty to thirty minutes is all it takes. But full disclosure: There are few things worse in life (at least in those moments) than stepping on something like a thorn or sharp rock that just causes your body to instantly recoil in pain! Scope out where you plan to walk first so you know what you'll be walking on. But in my experience, the rewards far outweigh the risk, and for that reason I continue to go on barefoot walks as often as I am able. Especially on my recovery days.

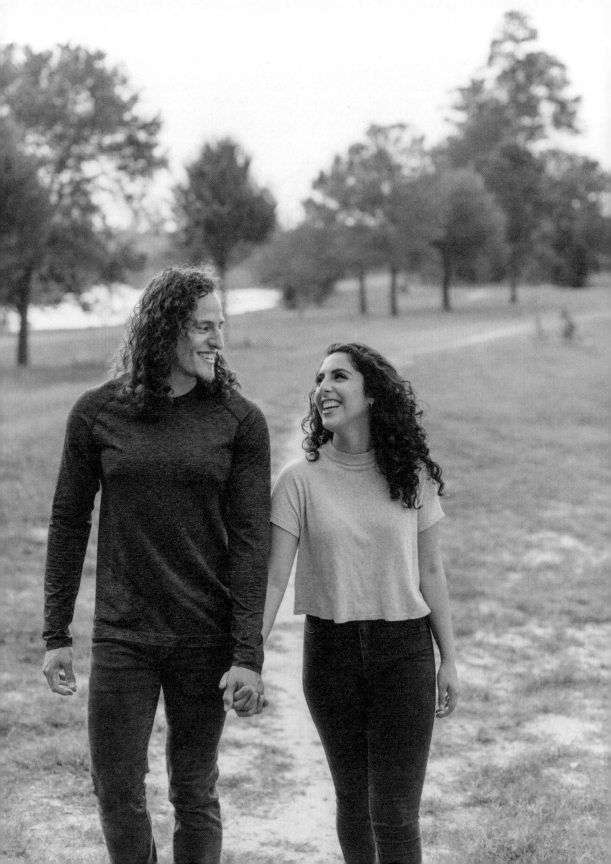

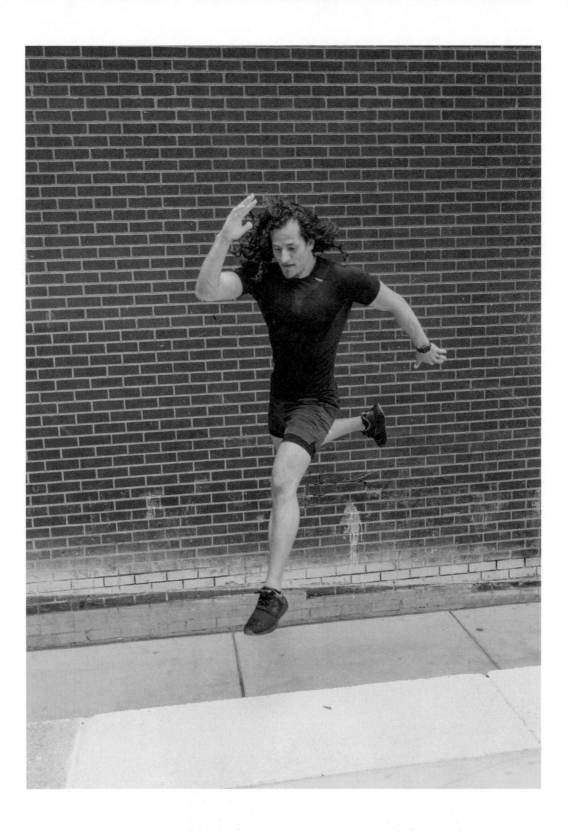

6

NUTRITION

Bottom line, if you put good in, you get good out. But of course the question is, "What is good?" This is a question I ask myself regularly. Is what's good for *you* good for *me*? Allergies, health conditions, and vitamin deficiencies vary from person to person, so what's perfect for you may not be what's perfect for me, and vice versa. There's vegan, paleo, keto, ancestral, carnivore, kosher, homestead, and many other diet plans out there that people live their lives by and that help them reach their health goals.

Here is what I generally ask in order to decide what's good: Where does it come from, and what's inside of it? Who made it, and what is its origin? What is its purpose? Is it fuel I can use for my machine of a body, or is it designed to make someone else rich by making people addicted to it or making it cheap enough to be wildly popular? There's a reason why elite athletes spend a lot of time and effort (and sometimes money) on nutrition. I tell people simply to take ownership of their health and begin the journey of educating themselves about nutrition.

I also try to take notice of how I feel after eating certain foods so I can recognize how they affect me. One example: As much as I love baked sweet potatoes, they always mess me up. Another example: As good as milkshakes taste, they always leave me with regret. When I crave those particular tastes, I replace them with sweet potato fries and ice cream instead, or other similar foods that I can eat without the negative side effects.

I'm a creature of habit. I'll gladly eat the same food every single day for weeks or months at a time without ever feeling a need to change it, especially if I'm getting what my body needs and seeing good results. Abby . . . not so much. My wife loves variety when it comes to food! But like everything else in our marriage, we strive to find a healthy balance and compromise.

Portion control is another huge problem, in my opinion. American portion sizes are insane compared to most other countries. In most cases, we're taking in way more than we need. I believe that strength comes from within and is an inside-out job. Our muscles can grow and improve only when they're well-nourished. Most adults need between 1,500 and 2,000 calories a day. For athletes, this number can increase by 500 to 1,000 more calories. Consult your doctor about your or your child's nutrition needs. They can help you determine a healthy daily calorie count. Over time, you will learn how to balance your intake and output to avoid extreme weight gain or loss.

Strength, like anything else, grows when fed and nourished correctly. And again, it takes time.

REGARDING ENERGY POWDERS

Some people use energy powders or pre-workout supplements to get hyped for their workout. I just add a high-quality warm-up to feel hyped for every workout. On that note, I have never used pre-workout powders of any kind, but I do understand that some people's lifestyles, workloads, and sleep schedules require a little extra stimuli for their workouts. That's fine too. Just make sure you also warm up properly.

Supplementation

I use what many consider to be a standard supplementation routine including zinc, vitamin D-3, and vitamin C. But over the last two years

I also began using collagen supplements. I have seen a huge improvement in my physical recovery from training. Collagen has been shown to improve elasticity and even help with gut health.

Hydration

I aim to drink half my body weight in ounces of water each day, not counting other liquids. Water is the first thing I put into my body after I wake up. I drink twelve to sixteen ounces of water with each meal, and I end my day with a small glass after I've hit my goal.

FASTING

I practice intermittent fasting regularly, where after an early dinner I won't eat again until midafternoon the next day—usually sixteen to eighteen hours between meals. It's proven very efficient on my rest days. It's one of my more recent practices, and I'm seeing great results in my overall health and well-being. This has been shown to reduce inflammation and helps us really maximize what we're putting into our bodies for recovery.

Even with these good habits, I learned a lesson about hydration the hard way. With the duration of active movement and level of sweat that I was releasing during my daily workouts, I began experiencing dehydration and didn't understand how that could be! How could I be drinking so much water and still be dehydrated? My muscles were overly sore, my body felt seriously fatigued, and my muscles would even cramp up during my workouts. That is not how anyone wants to feel after a great workout and *definitely* not if you're training as a pro in your sport! Live and learn, I guess.

Now, in addition to drinking half my body weight in ounces of water each day, during my hard workouts I always have at least sixteen ounces of an electrolyte drink in a second water bottle because I know I'm going to be sweating a lot. Bottom line: Hydration is key! I don't have those problems anymore, and neither should you!

My go-to drink after an intense workout where I sweat a ton is . . . pickle juice! After my "leg day" training where I do high-intensity interval sprinting,

I drink some pickle juice to prevent cramping or alleviate cramping if it has already begun.

Also, my first drink each day is sixteen ounces of water with an added mineral supplement. Stay hydrated, my friends!

Protein

At least once a day—sometimes twice on more intense training days—I'll use a standard shaker bottle and have vanilla almond milk mixed with chocolate bone broth protein powder. Collagen protein helps strengthen tendons and can improve muscle and joint interaction in athletes, which is critical for my sport. Bone broth has lots of vitamins and amino acids, and can actually help strengthen your bones and guard against injury.

Treats

I'm not an ascetic when it comes to my diet! God gave us good things to enjoy, and I like to enjoy chocolate almost every day because it makes me happy!

Vanilla almond milk is my go-to drink other than water. I use it with my smoothies, shakes, and cereals.

I love berries of all kinds—including berries that have been dipped in dark chocolate! Fruits and lightly salted nuts taste great and are healthy, nutrient-rich snacks. I'm still working on vegetables by themselves (nobody's perfect!), but as long as they're sautéed, I love them as sides with my dinner.

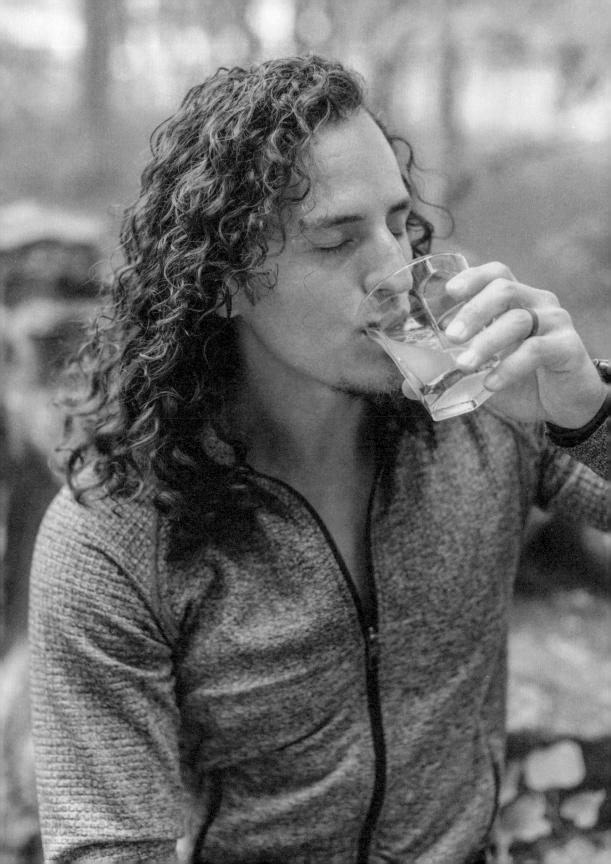

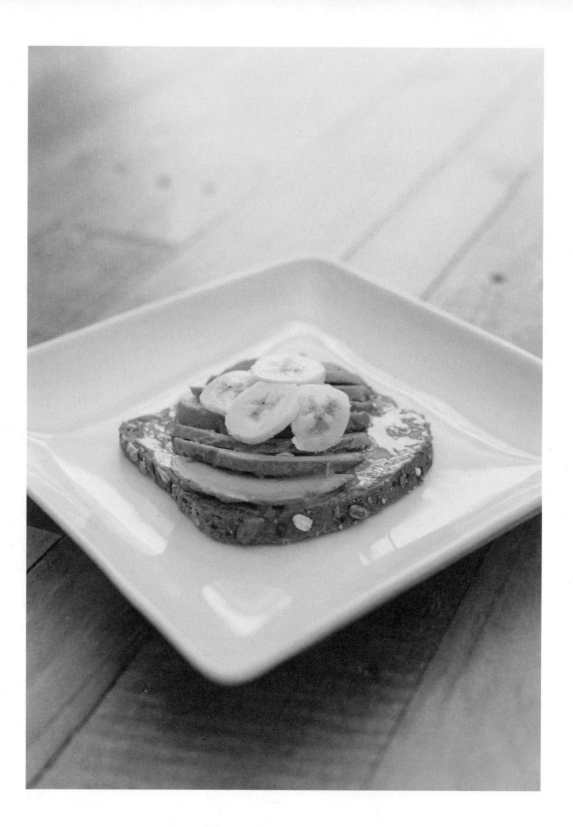

Peanut Butter, Avocado, and Banana Sandwich

I love sandwiches. They are a good (and quick) source of protein, carbs, and calories, all of which athletes need. Egg, turkey, ham, peanut butter and jelly—it doesn't matter to me! The key is to not overthink it.

Serving size: 1

1 slice whole grain bread
1 T. natural peanut butter
½ banana, sliced
½ avocado, sliced

1. I like to toast the bread first, but you can skip this step if you prefer.

2. Spread the peanut butter on the slice of bread.

3. Add the banana and avocado slices.

Avocado Toast

Serving size: 1

½ avocado
Lime juice, to taste
Paprika, to taste
Salt and pepper, to taste
1 tsp. cilantro, chopped
1 large egg, fried to taste
1 slice whole grain bread

1. In a small bowl, combine the avocado, lime juice, paprika, salt, and pepper, and mash them together with a fork. Stir in the cilantro.

2. Heat a small nonstick skillet over medium heat. Coat the surface of the pan with cooking spray, crack your egg into a bowl, and then drop the egg into the pan. Season it with salt and pepper. Let the egg cook to your desired level, flipping the egg if you prefer.

3. Toast the bread. Top your toast with the avocado mixture and then the egg. Garnish with a little extra cilantro and paprika.

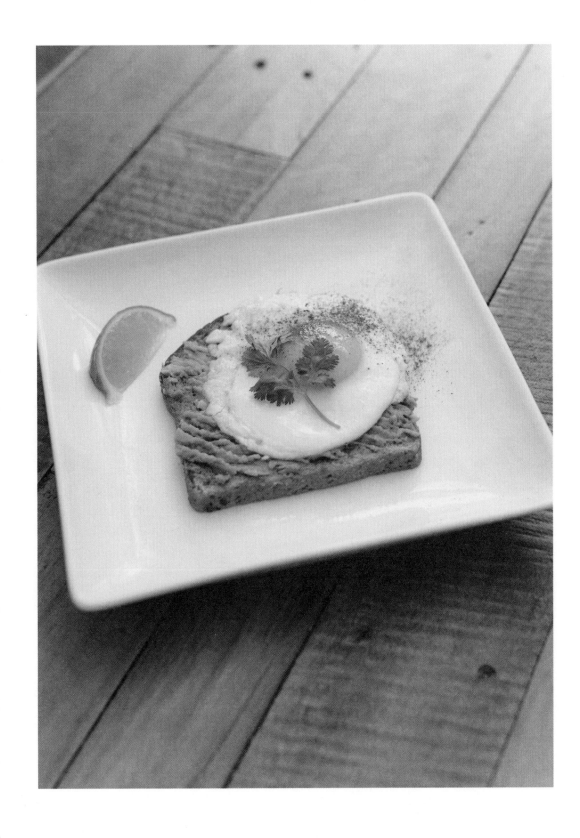

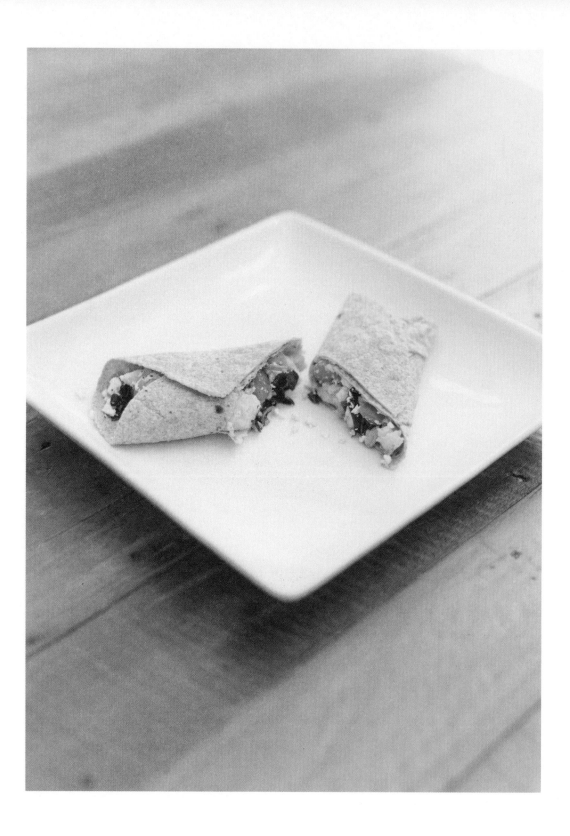

Spinach and Egg Wrap

Wraps are quick and easy to make, they are easy to transport, and they are good sources of protein, carbs, and nutrient-rich veggies. And they won't break the bank! They don't take long to prepare and are a great alternative to cheap, additive- and preservative-saturated fast food.

Serving size: 1

½ cup spinach, chopped
2 eggs, beaten
Large wrap or tortilla
¼ cup feta cheese
½ tomato, diced
Salt and pepper, to taste

1. Heat a skillet over medium heat. Coat the surface with cooking spray.

2. Sauté the spinach until it wilts. Add the eggs and scramble them with the spinach for about 2 minutes. You may also want to warm your tortilla in a separate skillet at the same time.

3. Transfer the eggs and spinach mixture to the warm tortilla. Top with the cheese, tomato, salt, and pepper. Fold the edges of the tortilla over the filling.

Turkey and Cucumber Wrap

Serving size: 1

Large wrap or tortilla

1 T. hummus

2 ounces turkey, sliced

1 or 2 slices of Provolone cheese

¼ cucumber, sliced in strips or match sticks

Red onion, sliced, to taste

Salt and pepper, to taste

1. Spread the hummus on the wrap or tortilla.

2. Top with turkey, cheese, cucumber, and onion. Season to taste.

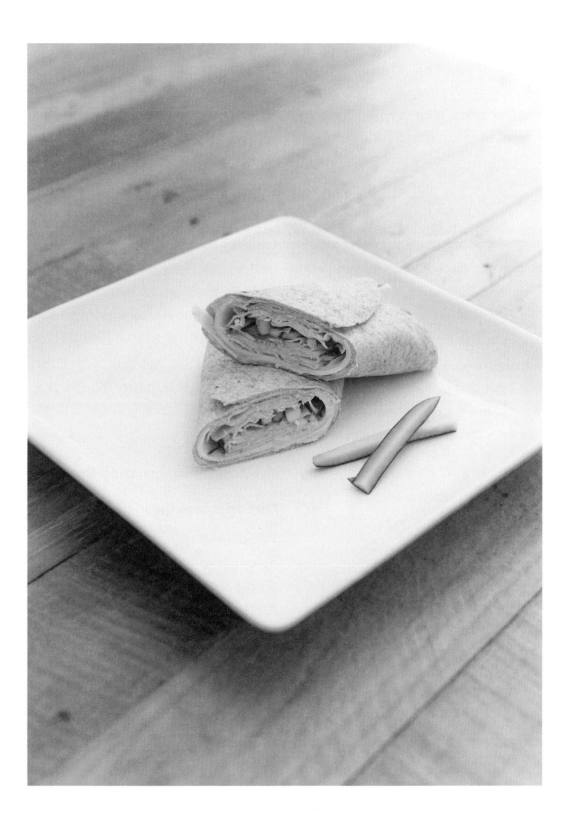

Rice bowls

Beef, chicken, shrimp—it's all amazing when it's in a rice bowl. Here are a couple of my favorite variations.

Poke Bowl

This is one of my favorite meals because it's so simple and full of good things. It's also a great meal to share with people. I lay out all the ingredients, charcuterie style, and let everyone build their bowls with what they like. If you think about it, poke bowls are kind of like deconstructed sushi: They use the same ingredients, but they are mixed up in a bowl and you can eat them with a fork. (Or chopsticks, if you're cool. I'm not that cool.) Vary the ingredients and amounts to best feed you or your guests. *See instructions below for preparing your ingredients.*

Sushi rice
Sushi-grade ahi tuna
Salt, pepper, sesame seeds
Cucumber, sliced
Carrot, shredded
Edamame, shelled
Broccoli, cut into small florets
  and blanched

Red onion, sliced thin
Avocado, peeled and cut into cubes

Optional toppings:

Wasabi soy
Spicy mayo
Sweet soy
Pickled ginger

Preparation

SUSHI RICE: This is a special type of short-grain rice that you can buy at most grocery stores. To prepare, first rinse your rice really, really well in a fine-mesh strainer, stirring it around with your fingers as you rinse it. The water will look cloudy at first (that's all the extra starch you're washing away) and

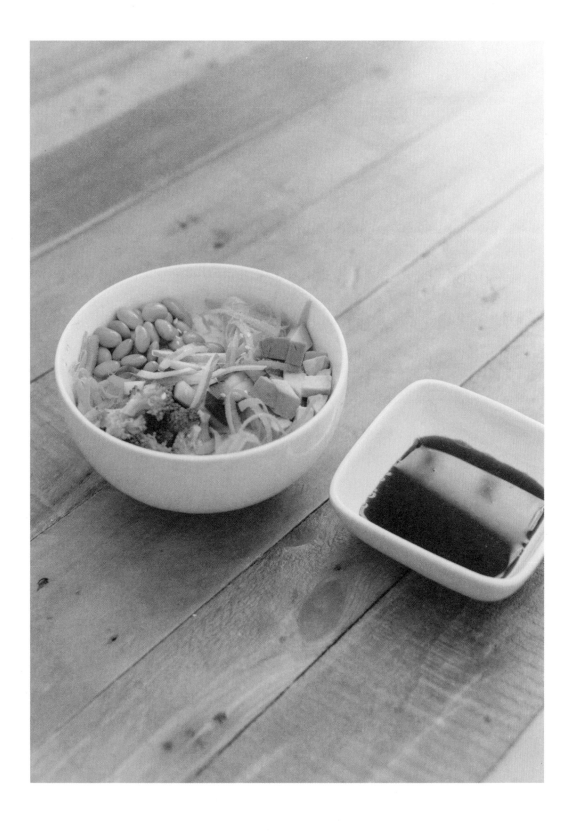

will eventually run clear. Cook the rice according to the package directions (usually 1½ cups rice with 2 cups water, cooked for 20 minutes). After the rice is cooked, you can season it with 2 tablespoons of white sugar and 1 teaspoon of salt dissolved in 2 tablespoons of rice vinegar. Drizzle the liquid mixture onto the hot rice while you are stirring it. Alternately, you can use any type of rice, seasoned or not, including brown rice, or skip the rice entirely.

AHI TUNA: Make sure you have sushi-grade ahi tuna! Season both sides of the raw tuna with salt and pepper. You can sprinkle on a thick crust of sesame seeds too if you want. Heat a little oil in a skillet over medium-high heat. Sear the tuna for 2 to 3 minutes on each side. I like it nice and rare and red in the center, with just a tiny rim of sear on the outside, but you can cook it the way you want. (Just don't complain to me when it is dry and tasteless if you are afraid to eat it rare.) Once the fish is cooked the way you want, slice it thinly across the grain. Alternately, you can use any kind of cooked fish you want, or cocktail shrimp, or even cooked chicken.

VEGGIES: This is where it gets really fun. I've suggested my personal favorite veggies and ways to prepare them, but you can change it up however you want. The more different veggies you invite to the party, the better it will taste, and you'll have more nutritional variety! Fresh herbs like cilantro, basil, and even dill would be great, and some people like to add fruit like mango or pineapple.

SAUCES: Again, you can get creative here! If there's a sauce you like on your sushi, it would probably be great with poke. Wasabi soy is easy to make: Just mix a little wasabi paste into some soy sauce or coconut aminos. Same with spicy mayo: Mix sriracha and mayo to the spiciness level you like. I buy sweet soy sauce at the Asian market, and you can probably buy lots of other interesting sauces there too. You could add other toppings as well, like fried onions, crushed peanuts, tempura flakes, or pickled ginger.

Chipotle Bowl

This is another great meal to share, and you can make it as complicated or simple as you like. Use the parts of the recipe that you like and skip the parts you don't. It's pretty much all optional.

Cumin rice
Chipotle chicken
Charro veggies
Guacamole
Salsa or pico de gallo
Tortilla chips
Cheese
Sour cream

CUMIN RICE: Thoroughly rinse 1½ cups basmati rice in a fine-mesh strainer until the water runs clear. Meanwhile, melt some butter in a saucepan and toast 1 teaspoon of cumin seeds for about a minute, until you can smell it. Add your rinsed rice and toast it for 2 to 3 minutes, stirring occasionally. Add 2¼ cups water, 1 teaspoon salt, and a bay leaf, then stir and cover. When it comes to a boil, turn the heat down to low and cook for 17 minutes, then remove the pan from the heat. Let it stand, covered, a few minutes, then remove the bay leaf and serve. You can use any type of rice in your bowl or even skip the rice altogether.

CHIPOTLE CHICKEN: Cut 1½ to 2 pounds of boneless, skinless chicken breasts or thighs into bite-size chunks (I like to use a mix of both light and dark meat). In a small bowl, make your seasoning mixture using 2 teaspoons of kosher salt and ½ teaspoon of each of the following: ground cumin, chili powder, coriander, chipotle pepper, garlic powder, smoked paprika, and black pepper. Sprinkle the seasoning mix all over your chicken pieces, rub it

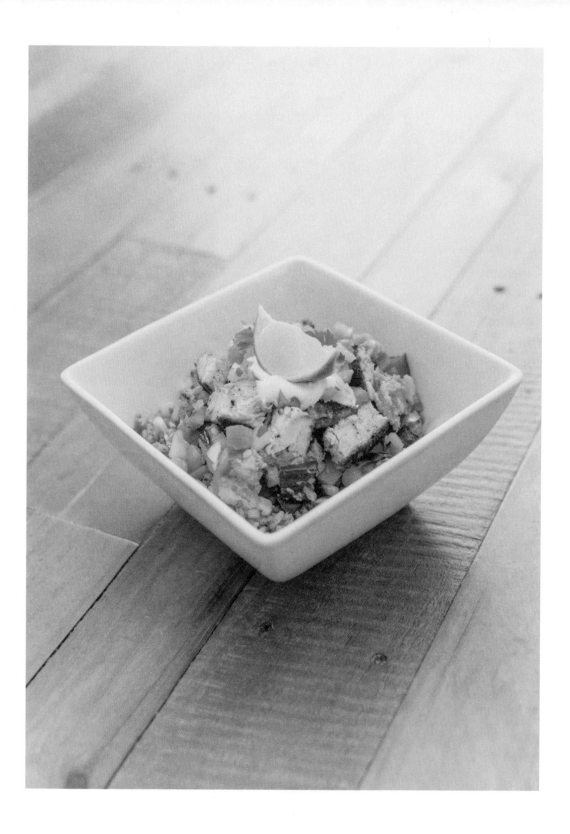

in a little, and then cook the meat in a really hot skillet, stirring occasionally, until the chicken is cooked through. (Don't crowd your skillet. You may need to cook this in 2 or 3 batches to give the chicken room to cook evenly.)

CHARRO VEGGIES: You can use whatever veggies you want. Some great options are onions, whole garlic cloves, bell peppers, poblano peppers, zucchini, and fresh corn cut off the cob. Cut the onions and peppers into bite-size pieces and toss them together on a roasting pan with some whole garlic cloves, a drizzle of olive oil, and a sprinkle of salt and chipotle powder. Roast in a convection oven at 400° for 10 to 12 minutes, until the edges are a little charred and the veggies are as soft as you like. You can add the zucchini and fresh corn to the pan with the other veggies and roast them all together or roast the zucchini and corn separately (or add them in later) since they do cook at different rates. It's tricky to get zucchini to char but not be mushy; the best way I've found is to cut it into thick planks, NO salt or oil, and roast it at a really high heat in a pan lined with parchment paper (so it doesn't stick). If you don't mind mushy zucchini, throw it in with the other veggies.

GUACAMOLE: Cut good, ripe avocados in half and scoop the flesh into a bowl. Mash it up with a fork and add a squeeze of lime juice and a good sprinkle of kosher salt. You can jazz it up with a little finely diced onion and cilantro, or even some raw tomato. The only way to screw it up is to have bad avocados. If the avocados are ripe, it will taste great no matter what you add!

Everyone can build a bowl to their own preference with rice, chicken, and vegetables mixed together in the bowl and topped with guacamole, salsa or pico de gallo, your favorite cheese, and sour cream. Serve with tortilla chips.

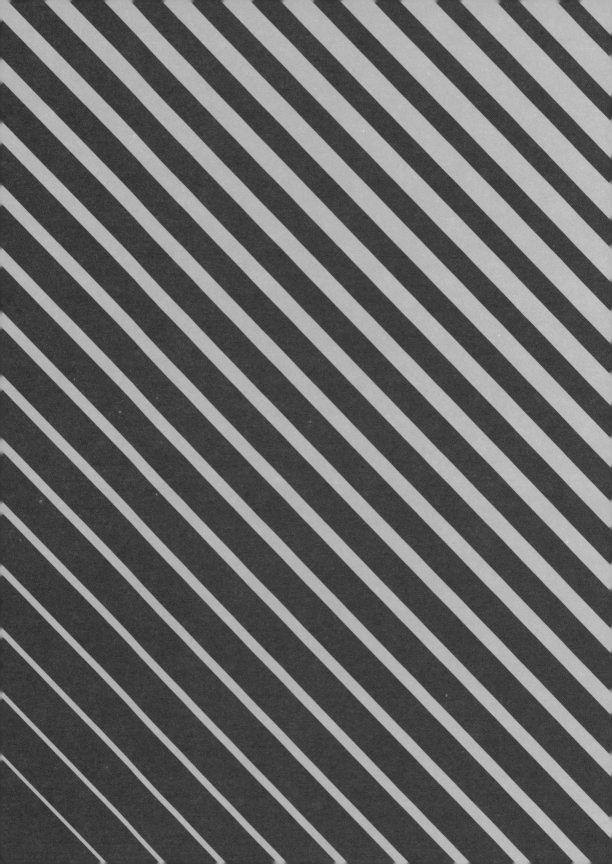

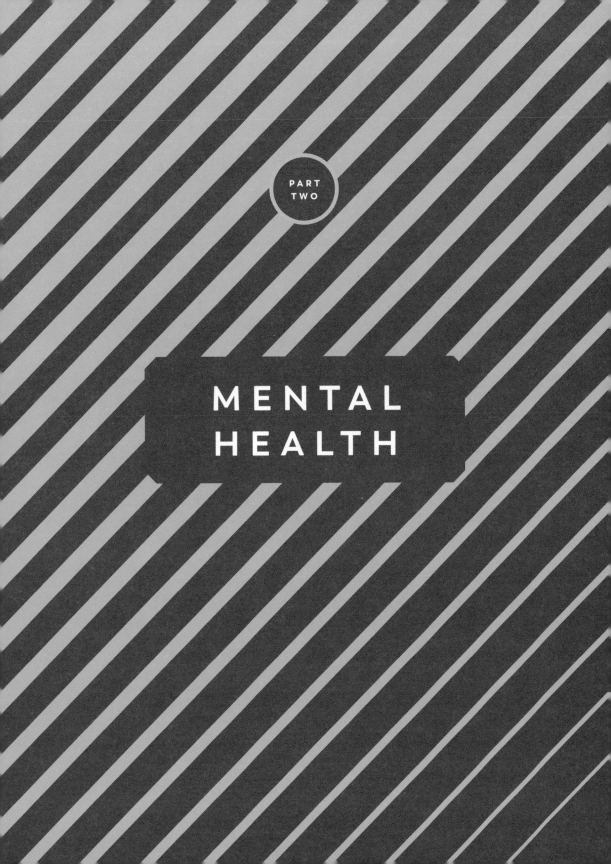

PART
TWO

MENTAL
HEALTH

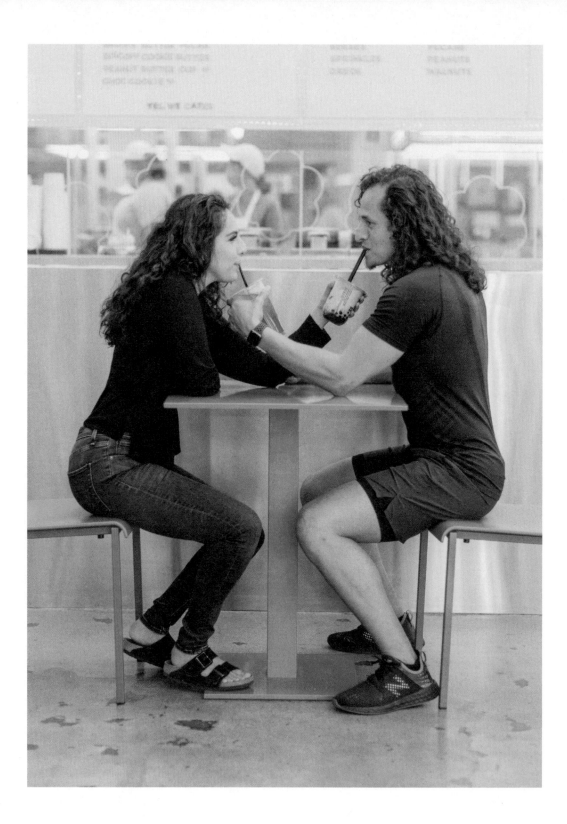

WHOLISTIC HEALTH

Mental health is crucial to living a wholistically healthy life. Being able to focus during a competition helps me avoid mistakes that could cause me to lose crucial seconds on a course—or even worse, cause severe injury. Mind and body are connected, and an unhealthy mind can affect more than just performance. Those who are anxious and stressed all the time can be more likely to develop heart disease and other problems.

I'm pretty good at not letting huge issues and problems affect my life and peace . . . but the *little* things can really add up over time and hit me hard when I'm not expecting it. When too many seemingly insignificant things happen at once, they can really mess with me.

When it comes to mental health and wellness, these are some of the many things I do on a semi-regular basis to keep me grounded.

Accountability Is Key

I've given a few people full access to my life. One of my most crucial mental health habits is to have open and fully transparent conversations with these loved ones. In the church, we call this accountability, but I think it's also just wise practice.

I'm very much a people pleaser. That can be very taxing and lead to a lot of over-commitment. I can burn myself out if I'm not careful. I realize that I need to limit the things I say yes to, but it is hard to do because I don't want anyone to dislike me! However, saying yes for the wrong reasons can lead to burn-out and resentment. As I assess the gifts the Lord has given me and the doors He has opened, I also make space in my life to consider some of the downsides of those opportunities and of my character.

I have people in my life who aren't yes-men and who call it as they see it. They can be honest and truthful without having an agenda. Therapists can be people like that. They can help us navigate who we are and who God has made us to be.

I have my own group of "counselors" with whom I can share in a safe place. They help me put one foot in front of the other, and they also help me run to the Lord. These are people like my wife, my parents, my mentors, and my pastors. Like everything else in life, having a healthy mind requires an intentional process.

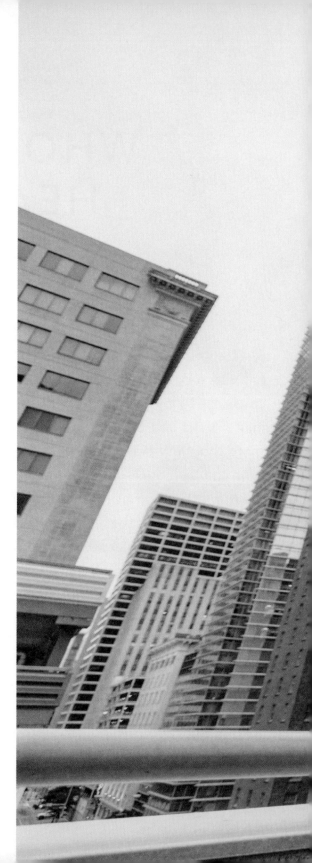

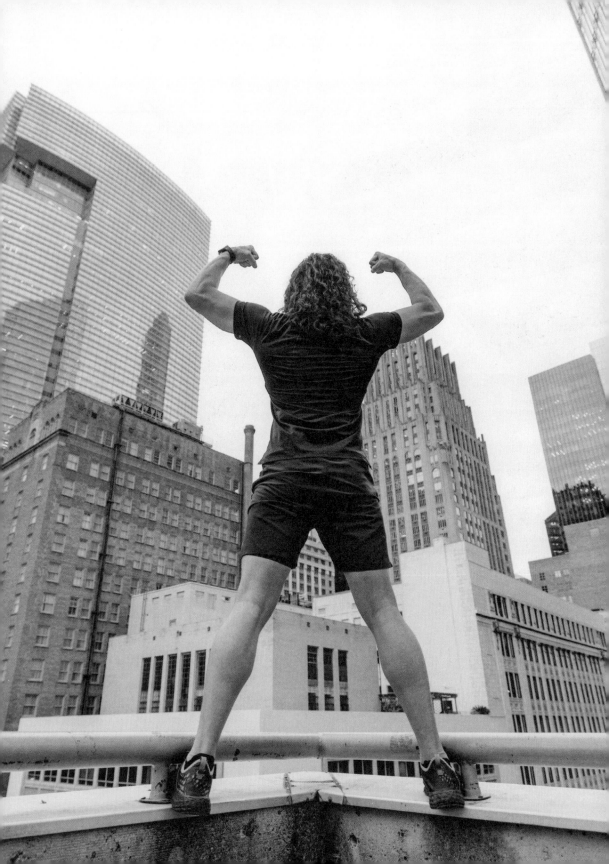

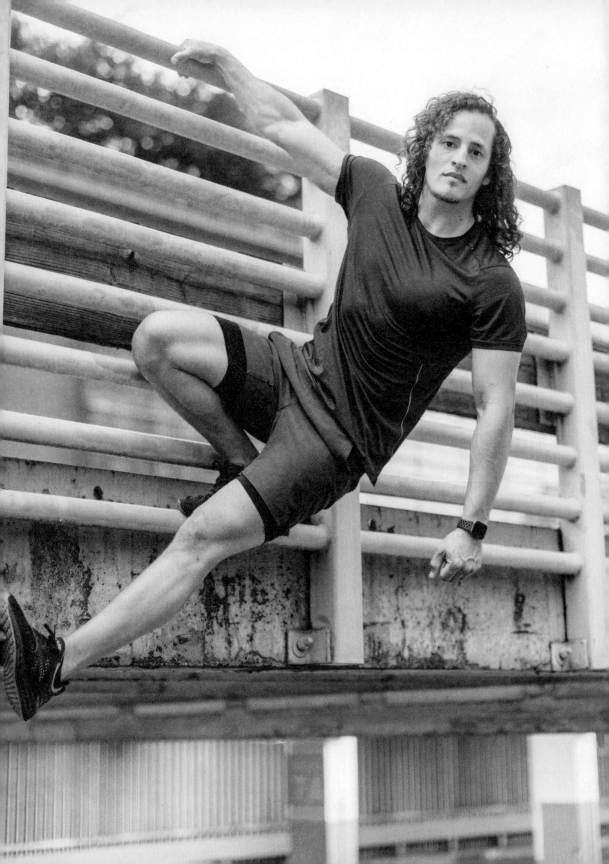

Not All Anxiety Is Bad Anxiety

I've wrestled with anxiety my whole life. When I realized that anxiety and excitement are two sides of the same coin, I finally began to understand anxiety and harness its power. My body reacts to excitement the same way it reacts to anxiety, so I sometimes confuse the two. When I first picked up the phone to ask Abby on a date or first stepped on the stage for a competition—those were *good* things! But the world sometimes says that all anxiety is bad.

Some studies indicate that our bodies can't tell the different between anxiety and excitement. In 2015, as I looked at a course I was about to run for the first time, my heart started pounding and my legs started trembling. I began to pray, talking it out with the Lord. He is a friend who sticks closer than a brother, the God of all comfort. I asked, *Lord, how do I get through this?* Whatever the outcome, I gave Him the results. As I did, I experienced a noticeable change in my mind. My hands were still trembling, but the fear and anxiety turned into an excitement that I'd never felt before. My perspective had shifted.

I'm also a thrill seeker, and I realized that the course would be a thrill for me. So all I focused on was the obstacle right in front of me. I experience a kind of euphoria every time I run a course. At every round, more is at stake. It's easy for me to look at negative consequences if I fail, but I need to remind myself of my reason for being there and my purpose in life. I'm not always perfect at keeping that perspective, and I need to have people in my corner keeping me on my mental game. I need to consistently assess my perspective in the moment and not live off yesterday's successes.

Meditation and Breathing

Meditation is an interesting topic in today's culture. With the increasing public spotlight on mental health, meditation has become more popular. However, some people still seem to be conflicted about it because of its historic link to various religions or new age beliefs. For some people, this topic can be very polarizing.

Meditation for me is simply focusing on my breathing, focusing on my goals, or talking with God.

I often take time in my busy day to focus on my breathing and use different exercises I've learned over the years to refocus and calm down. As a choir kid and vocalist for half of my life, I learned many diaphragmatic breathing exercises and routines to help maximize my singing ability. Those routines stuck with me, and I still take the time to breathe slowly and intentionally for a minute or two multiple times in any given day.

Ever have someone tell you to chill out and "take a deep breath"? Well, I remind myself to do that daily. I also love to stretch, and as an athlete you need to focus specifically on your breathing while stretching in order to relax as much as possible and get the maximum benefits of those stretches. If you don't relax into the stretch, you may force your muscles to go beyond their healthy limits, which will cause even greater soreness the next day.

In my meditation and breathing practices, I'm not trying to empty myself of who I am, and I'm not chanting a mantra to transcend this reality and reach a higher spiritual state of being. I'm just hitting the brakes on my bullet train of a life. A few minutes of intentional breathing will lower my heart rate and help me focus and clear my head.

Sometimes I'll do "box breathing," which was made popular by the Navy SEALs. You take a slow, deep breath, counting to four while you breathe in. Then you hold for four seconds, breathe out for four seconds, and hold for another four seconds. It's a four-by-four ratio that can help you stay relaxed and alert.

You can use various active breathing patterns and recovery breathing patterns in different scenarios, like sprints or marathons. Many of my friends love the Wim Hof method, in which you get comfortable, close your eyes, clear your mind, and take thirty to forty deep breaths. You exhale your last deep breath and hold until you need to breathe again.

One exercise I use nightly for falling asleep is "climbing up a ladder" with my breathing—filling and emptying my diaphragm and upping the ratio by one pull and push of air each time. Two deep inhales, two exhales; three inhales, three exhales; all the way up to ten or more, then back down. I do that most nights while lying in bed right before praying and going to sleep.

Usually when I meditate and breathe, I also pray and dream with God. I have learned that as a Christian, I hear the Lord speak more clearly when I just stop, breathe, and listen. The Bible says, "Be still, and know that I am God" (Psalm 46:10). Sometimes all we need to do is pump the brakes, breathe, and listen for what He wants to say to us. I've gotten many "God ideas" while doing just that. I will also breathe and meditate on the Word of God, focusing on whatever passage or verse of Scripture He has been using to speak to me.

My mentality as a person and as an athlete has a lot to do with the time I spend practicing intentional breathing and meditating on who I

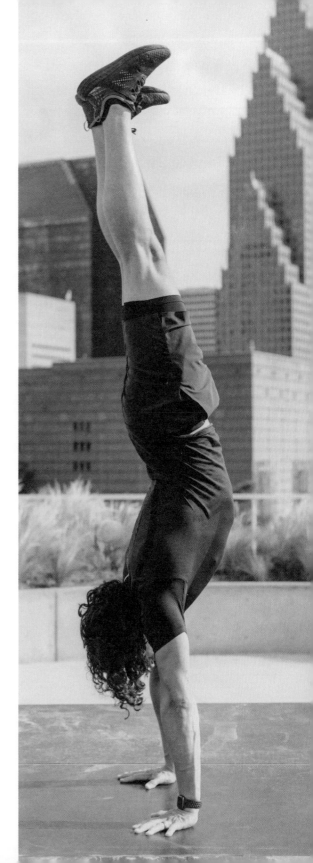

am and whose I am. This practice—focusing on my breathing and meditating on all the Lord has done for me and what I believe He's still yet to do with my life—sort of bulletproofs my mental state of trusting in a good God who has good plans that I get to be a part of. Bad days don't affect me as long or as painfully because my mind is set on other things. And this discipline doesn't take any more than a couple of minutes each day.

Yawning

I've become known as the guy who yawns. People in the ninja community and media have joked, "He's so strong, the course is putting him to sleep!" When I used to compete vocally, the competitions always seemed to be early in the morning, and I would naturally yawn. I would be so nervous that my heart would pound out of my chest, and I'd take short, erratic breaths. It was borderline hyperventilation due to stress even though I was prepared and should have felt confident. But I began to realize that after a nice, long, deep yawn, I always felt so much better and my heart rate would calm down a bit. I've heard that our brains can't tell the difference between a real and a fake yawn. I feel like living proof of that theory.

When I'm freaking out or I just really need to focus, I take a big, deep yawn, and then I feel ready to go. To this day, I'll do that in between obstacles when needed. It helps with my breathing and any intimidation that might be coming from a sketchy new obstacle. I've become very, very good at doing what needs to be done in the heat of the moment by controlling my breathing.

I have to constantly remind myself to breathe. God designed our bodies with breathing turned on "auto," and it can be surprisingly difficult to switch our breathing to "manual." Ninja athletes sometimes do one or two obstacles, dismount, and then take a huge gasp of air because they *stopped breathing*. It's understandable—you have to complete a dynamic

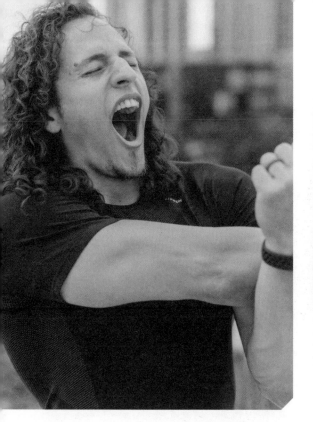
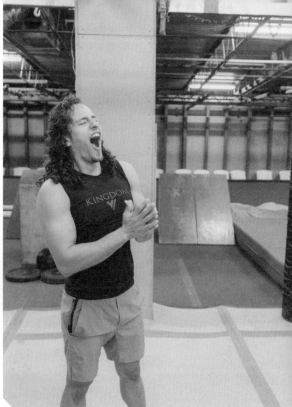

course without ever having tried it before. Plus, it's high impact and high cardio! There's already a lot to think about, so it's easy to put focused breathing on the back burner of your mind, even when you know better. What rings louder in your head is usually something like, *Don't let go! Don't fall!* But I had already used calming and breathing exercises for many years as a vocalist, and I just kept them up as a Ninja. It has had a huge effect on my competitions.

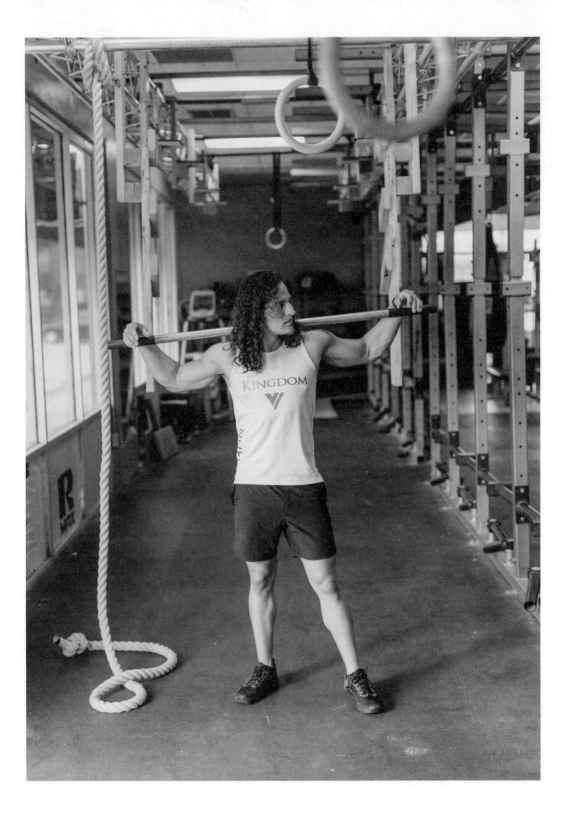

8

MOTIVATION

Through the combined influence of my family, my coaches, and my faith, I have learned to constantly stretch myself out of my comfort zone. Before tackling a difficult task, you have to train yourself to do it. Remember, it doesn't matter how much faith someone might have in you—if you don't have the will to get up and do it, then their faith in you won't matter.

So believe in yourself, start small, and work your way up to bigger things in life. Control what you can and daily try to step out of your comfort zone.

Growing up, anytime a mentor (or the Lord) asked me to do something I was scared to do, my heart rate would spike and anxiety would overwhelm me. But deep down I knew they saw something in me that I didn't, and I wanted to try even if I didn't know whether I was capable. It's very important to have people like that in your life. In high school, a friend of mine read *Do Hard Things* by Steve Magness. He and I challenged each other to never be complacent and to always push ourselves for the better.

I now try my hardest to step up to every challenge—both the physically and mentally demanding ones—give it my absolute best shot, and then trust God for the results. It doesn't always turn out the way I want it to, but the whole point really is just to stretch myself and give it my best effort. Either way, I always gain valuable information and instruction on how I need to grow in the future. With this growth mindset, I welcome the challenges, no matter how daunting.

Doing hard things physically also prepares me for other kinds of unexpected challenges in life. Things like cold showers, hot saunas, barefoot walks outside, and pushing my limits in workouts build habits into my life that push my limits and give me the mental fortitude I need in order to reach my goals as an athlete. Setting myself up to regularly overcome small inconveniences in life gives me the long-term benefits of a mentality that I won't back down from any challenge presented to me.

The Power of Self-Talk

Self-talk matters. I need to make sure that in my head and heart I'm not constantly putting myself down or cursing myself for making mistakes. As people often say, "Be careful what you tell yourself, because you're always listening." Learn to control your thought life. I encourage myself. Daily. The Bible even says David "strengthened himself in the LORD his God" when he was having more than just your average bad day and nobody was there to cheer him up (1 Samuel 30:6). You won't always have someone else to encourage and motivate you. You have to learn to do that for yourself when you need it the most. I regularly remind myself who I am and whose I am. I also remind myself of my dreams, goals, and purpose in life. On the good days and the bad days.

You have to be your own first line of defense against toxic thought patterns and unhealthy habits. Don't curse or put yourself down when you inevitably fall or fail, because the truth is, life happens. Now, don't go on the opposite end and begin making excuses either. Instead, hold yourself to your standards and core values and continue to aim higher. It's okay to stumble and fall as you make your way uphill. All of this takes place within your mind, and it can be a battleground at times.

The Bible says that "each heart knows its own bitterness, and no one else can fully share its joy" (Proverbs 14:10 NLT). Nobody else may fully understand what you've been through in life. You do. But while you look for others to process through those experiences with, have a filter that you use that leads you to a better place or simply keeps you in a good headspace. Remind yourself of the promises of God throughout Scripture—that though you fall you can get back up (Proverbs 24:16), that even what your enemies intended for evil God can use for good (Genesis 50:20), and that God has good plans for you, to give you hope and a future (Jeremiah 29:11).

Remember that the whispers you utter to yourself matter much more than the shouts of someone else toward you.

The mind is a powerful thing. And faith comes by hearing (Romans 10:17). If all you ever hear is "You'll never be good enough," or "Why bother trying; you could never do it . . . you won't make it," then even if it's a complete lie, you will accept it over time and even begin believing it yourself. But if you speak life and truth over yourself, your automatic response will be to reject the lies you may hear in your head about your memories or your present circumstances.

The Bible says to think about whatever is true, noble, just, pure, lovely, admirable, excellent, or praiseworthy (Philippians 4:8). Why? Because it will shift your worldview and have the most profound effects on your life and attitude—for the better.

We need to have courage. But to do that, we need to constantly be encouraged. And if that's not coming from others, then it definitely needs to be coming from within us. Be careful what you tell yourself, because you're always listening. So the next time you talk to yourself, make sure you end the conversation feeling a little better and more hopeful than when you began. Have good self-talk.

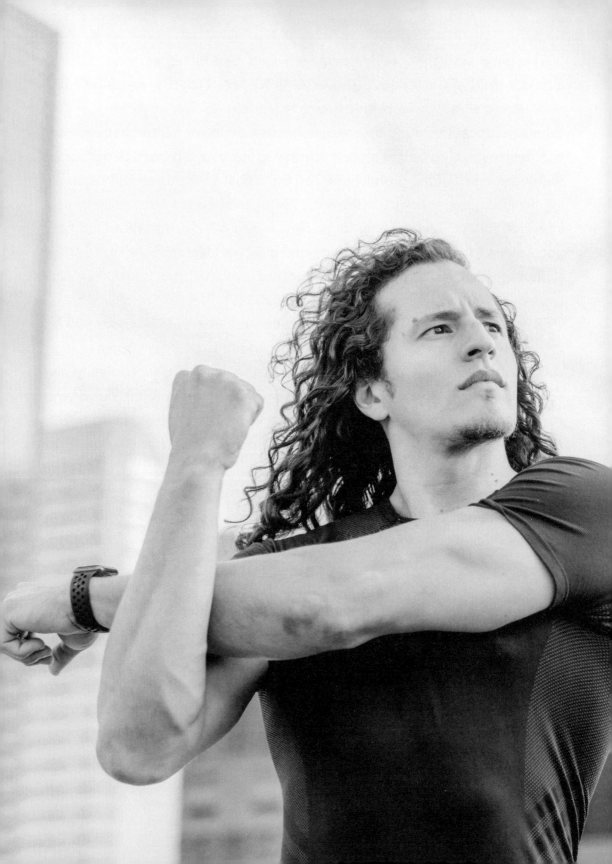

ANW SEASON 11: WATER WALLS, LAS VEGAS FINALS, STAGE 2, 2019

Water Walls was the last obstacle of stage 2 for seasons 10 and 11. You drop into a container of water and swim though a corridor while having to open up and swim through three different doors to get to the finish platform and buzzer. This was one of the most intense obstacles the show has ever had! Holding your breath while being physically exhausted and swimming through a tight space is one of the most demanding challenges I've faced on a ninja course. I didn't get a chance to attempt it in season 10, so when I did in season 11 it was incredible!

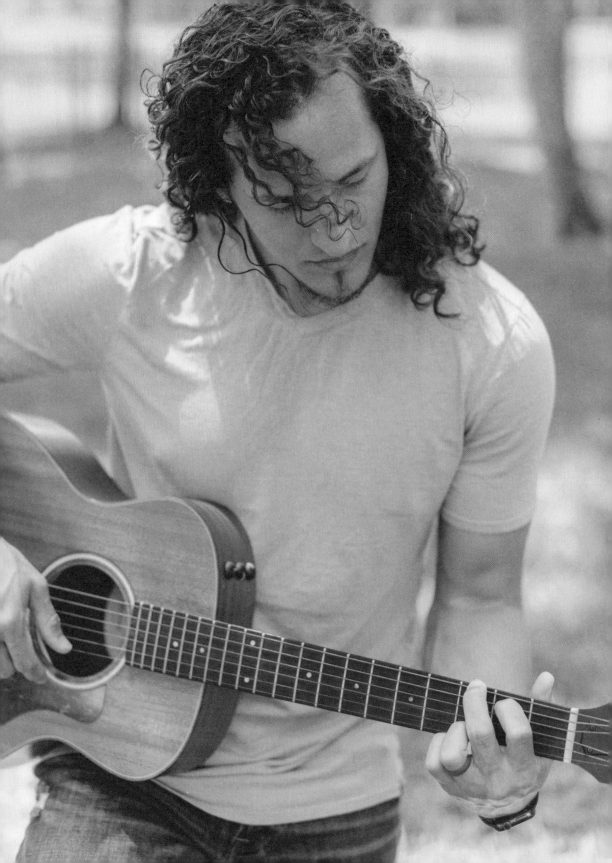

Music Motivator

I believe that music is one of the greatest gifts humanity has ever been given—instruments and voices, solos and ensembles, rhythms and dynamics, melodies and harmonies . . . music takes you places, and it's incredible the stories that you can tell using song. I love listening to many different genres of music and the creative distinctions that make them special. I enjoy classical, pop, hip-hop, rock, and even metal. There's something to appreciate in every style and creative expression of music. Regardless of the genre that I'm listening to, I believe that words carry weight—they have meaning and power behind them. I believe that God spoke the earth into existence and we, being image bearers of God, likewise carry a responsibility with the words we say.

The Bible says death and life are in the power of the tongue (Proverbs 18:21), so in addition to "Christian music," I listen to any music that has meaning to me and brings me life in some way. I've never much cared for the top hits on the radio because so many of them seem to have toxic meanings and messages. A song can be catchy and have great vocals or a great beat behind it and be mastered perfectly, but if the words I'm hearing are tearing me down and not in some way building me up, then I won't be adding it to my playlists.

For my training, I have at least fifteen different hip-hop, rock, and metal playlists that continue to grow each year. I look forward to each week when new music is released, and I get to enjoy the new sounds and material from my favorite artists. I'll find songs or albums that speak to me, and I'll play them on repeat for weeks on end until Abby can't stand it anymore! The cycle truly never ends with music. But as with everything else in my life, I am very intentional about what I put into my body. My ears are no exception.

Life Balance

I'm still working on balance in life. Working hard is important, but rest is just as important. Because of that, I try to be as intentional as I can with my time. I love writing down what my week looks like, and I try to schedule it beforehand as much as I can. Even still, life happens, and it's easy to stuff my days and weeks with too many things. Training. Coaching classes. Time with family and friends. Working on more projects than I have time for.

You have to be intentional about scheduling time for rest. It's easy to get burned out when we schedule every aspect of our lives and then fall behind because something unexpected comes up. You can also risk injury if you over-train, and it will affect your health if you're only running on adrenaline. Abby helps keep me balanced and accountable, and other people also have access to my life and help keep me on the right path that God has called me to.

MORE LIFE LESSONS FROM MY DAD

My dad is a very traditional, thick-accented Colombian man. He was an incredible top-level pro soccer athlete in Colombia. Three knee surgeries later, and after coming to America, he had to give up competing at a professional level. After he stopped playing, my dad cofounded a soccer club in Kingwood, Texas, and continued coaching for almost twenty years. He was a hero to many kids. Growing up, it seemed like everywhere I went people would recognize my dad and yell, "Hey, Coach Carlos!" I thought my dad was famous! He got a job in oil and gas to pay the bills for five kids, but it's not a job he enjoys. The greatest show of love is sacrifice, and he has done that for his family. My parents did (and continue to do) their best, and God has always taken care of the rest.

My identity with my dad was never based on performance. He didn't coach me often, but when he did, he pushed me hard. I was never the soccer player he was . . . which really bummed me out. I could never measure up to what I saw in him. But despite all that, he was always so supportive of me trying other sports and activities—even when I stopped playing soccer altogether in high school. He told me, "Enjoy your life. Try new things and do what you love." The older I get, the closer I become with my dad.

But at the same time, that doesn't mean I just eliminate every scenario where I might have to work hard. There are seasons when certain things will take priority, and you have to just press through them. A season of grind, a season of rest, a season to focus on this, a season to focus on that. Just keep that balance between hard work and restful stillness.

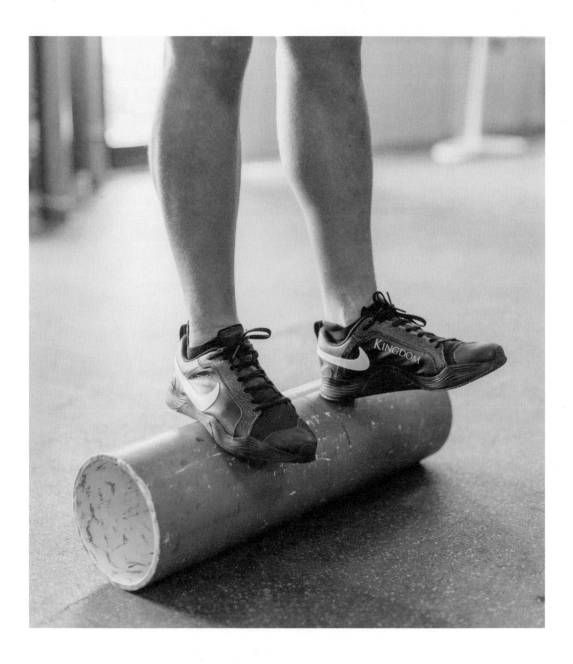

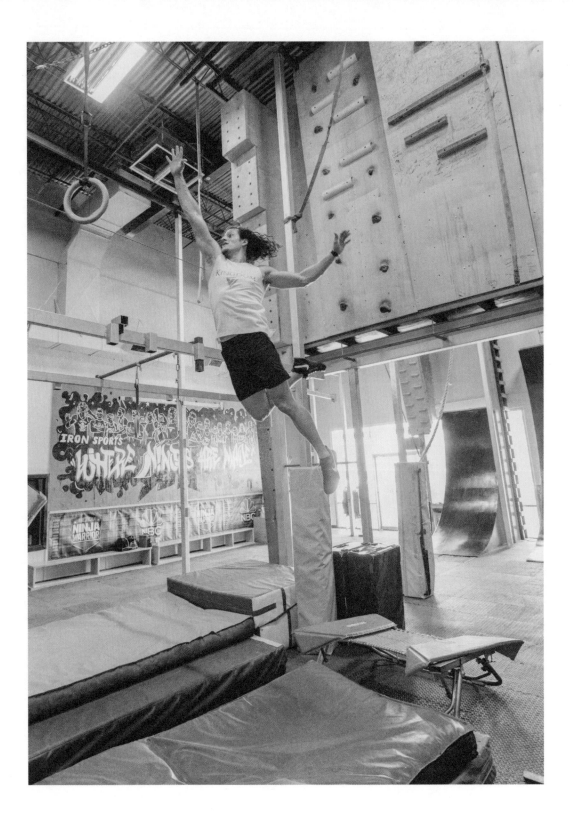

9

MINDSET

Passivity is a big obstacle in our culture, and it typically manifests when people feel so overwhelmed by options or so anxious about tasks that they just . . . sit . . . and wait for things to happen. I see this all over the culture now, as we have more options for distraction than ever before, and this distraction has detrimental results. But I also see it in my own heart, and I have experienced it firsthand too many times.

I often am more reactive than proactive, especially in the space of business. I'll sometimes wait for people to reach out or message me first rather than initiate a conversation. You only have a certain shelf-life or window of opportunity as an athlete, and I need to make sure I'm making the most of the moment I'm in.

My wife is business-minded in ways that I'm not. I thank God for that! She's efficient and organized, and I need her help in more ways than I ever knew! God has given me someone to pick up the slack where I lack the skills, and we make an incredible team.

Passivity is rooted in the fear of failure, and defeating it is rooted in a right relationship with failure. Because ninjas don't see the courses ahead of time, you have to trust yourself and your training and just attack the course with confidence. I see so many young people who are addled with fear of failure. They are afraid of being yelled at or reprimanded by a coach or parent . . . or perhaps they're afraid they can't live up to the expectations of others or even their own expectations for themselves. This fear keeps a lot of people stuck in life. When they come into the gym, they get to take joyful risks and learn to attack. They learn to be confident. This confidence can affect their attitude outside the gym as well.

You can overcome passivity only to the degree you understand that we are all human, and we all make mistakes, and we don't always win. Some of the best athletes walking this planet have experienced more failure than most people have ever even attempted. That was very freeing for me to learn. How many successful businessmen have lost it all, multiple times, before reaching the pinnacle they're at now? That gives me perspective for when I do fall and fail.

Losing does suck, so I don't downplay it. I hate it. I much prefer to win. (Did I mention I'm competitive?) Especially when I've put so much into something. It doesn't lessen the blow, but when you fail, you have to see the opportunity there to sharpen the sword you're working with. I have to want to do the activity more than I'm afraid to fail the activity.

It's fine and healthy to grieve losing, but you can learn from the loss and implement ways to prevent the same mistakes from happening again. When I was young, I would just try to forget about hard experiences as quickly as possible and run from them. I didn't want to reflect on my failures or open the door to them happening again, because it was so painful. This fear can keep us from all kinds of things—trying out for a sport, learning a new instrument, or picking up the phone to ask a girl out.

But now, by God's grace, I'm able to look at my disappointments and try to grow from them. Before, I wouldn't let myself go back to the moments of hurt and loss. But I saw that I was making the same mistakes over and over in life.

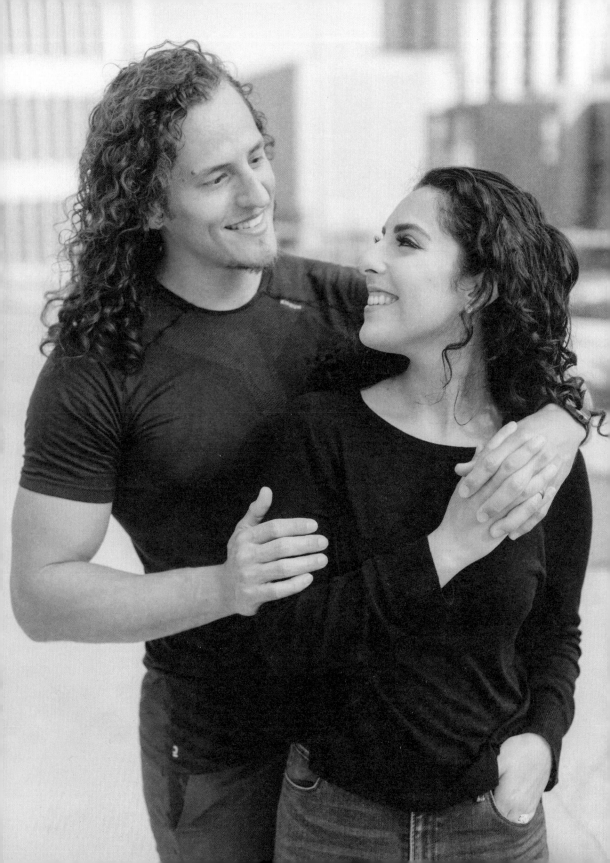

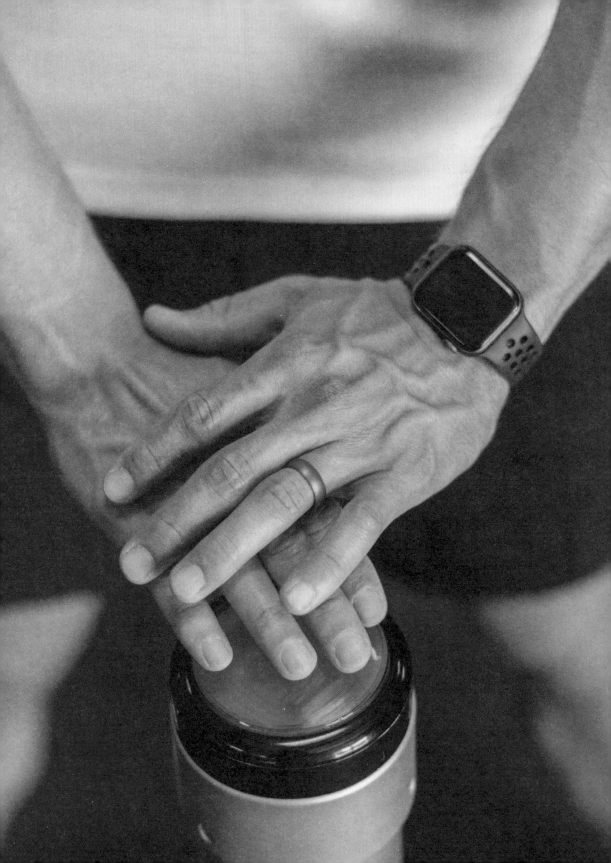

It's in those moments of looking back that we can really grow. Some of the best athletes I've been around see losses as almost more significant than victories. That's where you really see what you're made of and what is taking control of your heart.

Ninja Camaraderie

A unique aspect of this sport is how ninja is individualized. In early stages of competition and for so many years, if we all hit a buzzer, we're all moving on. Apart from the timed aspects of a competition, it's not really me versus you, it's us versus the course. I've found that I thrive in an individual setting more than in a group sport. Some people come alive in the lights, and I know for a fact that I'm one of them. It becomes my time to show up and show out, to do what I've prepared or practiced, and to give it everything I've got.

Even with the addition of the Power Towers and now head-to-head racing, there is still that sense of camaraderie and everybody is cheering everyone on! Each athlete is pushing themselves to the limits to see just how quickly they can complete the speed course. Still, the ultimate enemy is the course itself, and the individual pressure is on us to run like we never have before.

This is where the Hype. Gets. Real. It's where the rubber meets the road and all our hard work is put to the test. We understand the blood, sweat, and tears that go into training, and we want everyone to feel accomplished afterward, even if the results were not what they were hoping for.

It's interesting to think about how the audience sees the few minutes of the television competition but never knows the hours, weeks, months, and years of training that go into these course runs. Then there are the injuries, rehab, and grit that come with the territory of any sport and make comebacks that much harder and yet more meaningful. But the rest of us ninjas know. We know that if you fall early, you have to wait another year to try out again, just hoping you'll be selected to compete. So as fellow athletes, we try to help each other reach our potential, do our very best, and attain the results we've worked so hard to achieve.

Media and Technology

When it comes to mental health and the distractions that come from social media, gaming, subscription-based entertainment, and other technology available to us, it's not surprising to hear the ever-increasing statistics of people spending more time immersed in a fabricated reality than they do in the real world.

I'll be the first to admit I sometimes catch myself scrolling longer than I intended, bingeing more episodes than I meant to, or getting stuck reading the comments section. But for that reason, I approach all these digital distractions by monitoring and limiting my personal time spent on them. Like everything else in my life, self-discipline and creating healthy habits are vital to keeping something fun from consuming too much of my life.

My time is valuable, and I hate feeling like I wasted large portions

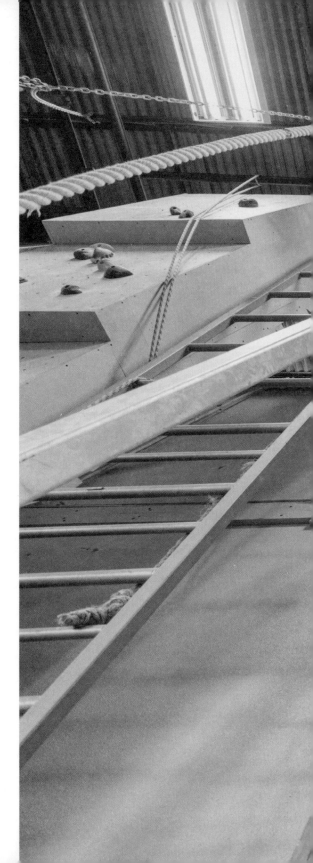

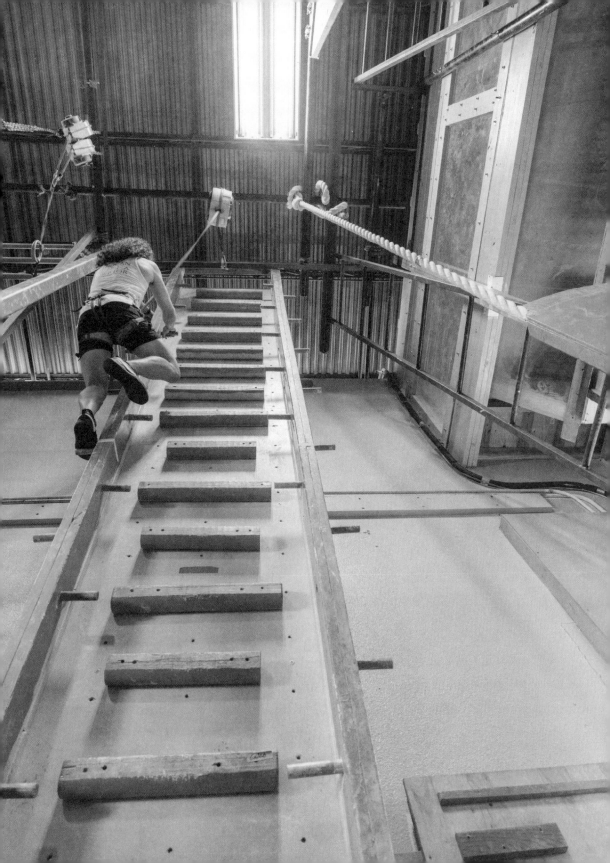

of it on a meaningless distraction. I acknowledge that these things are a part of my life and can be entertaining and even productive in moderation, but I can't let them dictate my life or derail my personal goals. I can't afford that, and I know that now more than ever before. With our free time, I believe we are either consuming or creating. The way we invest our free time really matters. I want to use my energy and free time creating something for myself and others rather than simply consuming that which doesn't truly benefit anybody in the long run.

So the next time you watch a show, follow that by reading a chapter of a book that helps you move forward in your life. Better yet, do something productive for half an hour first, and then reward yourself with an episode!

When you're scrolling through social media and see a family member or friend on your feed, give them a call and catch up for a bit.

We live in the age of influencers, and anyone can become famous online. But I prefer to focus on in-person events with tons of people rather than just posting something online. The time it takes to create content has never held much value to me when compared to spending time with people. And as a professional athlete, I only have so much free time in a day to pursue things other than my training.

If you follow me on social media, then you know I don't post all that much, probably to my detriment. I could have a lot more followers if I really tried. But that doesn't really matter to me. I love and appreciate those who do follow and support me. I'll get better at posting, but I'd always rather be having a meaningful conversation with someone, and that's what usually takes my free time.

There's a time and place for everything. Know what your priorities are, and don't let anything else in life distract you from them. Social media can be a great form of marketing and even a viable source of additional income. But it still costs you something.

Ninja PTSD

Mistakes and injuries are inevitable. Sometimes they can be very scary situations resulting in traumatic memory. Sometimes healing physically from an injury is the easy part, while healing mentally from it is a much different story. I've always encouraged people to get back up after falling, but sometimes you have to be more delicate and take things slower after a scary fall. You can see it in people's eyes, in their body language, and in their attempts to get back on the horse. Trauma happens, but walking through it with others can be especially helpful. Learning how to deal with trauma can take time and effort. And that's okay. My advice is to start small and work your way back up at your own pace using progressive training, increasing little by little your distances or heights or types of catches. You can get back to

JOURNALING

There are nights I try to fall asleep but stay awake for what feels like hours. I think of things I need to write down and address with the Lord—wrongs I have done toward Him or others and need to make right, or just insights and thoughts I've never had before and may never think of again. I keep a notebook handy for those moments. Whenever a thought pops into my head that I need to write down, I make a note. Often when I have a clear head, I'll think up nuggets of wisdom and truth.

Recently I thought of an insight related to a common struggle many men face. First John 2:16 talks about the lust of the flesh, the lust of the eyes, and the pride of life. Some men struggle with the lust of the flesh: I want her. Other men struggle with the lust of the eyes: I want that. And some men struggle with the pride of life: Look at what I've got. And yet none of these things are ever enough because of the toxic mindset they begin with.

I was able to use those sleepless moments to note the importance of finding ultimate satisfaction in God alone.

where you were before and even surpass the skills you once had. Learning to stop and recognize if you have any trauma-related stress associated with a specific obstacle is the first step to overcoming.

Injuries and Discouragement

Like most people, I often compare myself to others. Specifically, I see those who aren't injured and think about how hard it has been for me to work through certain injuries. If left unchecked, this thinking frustrates me to no end. Because I am so passionate about competing in my sport, an injury—even a minor one—*I hate it!* I hate those setbacks! I hate how easy it is to get injured, and I especially hate getting an injury that easily could have been prevented. After an injury, I look back and think, *Why did I even try that move in the first place?*

But life is not always fair, and you need to learn to roll with the punches. Now whenever I injure or "tweak" something, I try to find any other means to supplement my training without reinjuring or worsening the problem area. Often, even if I am injured, I still need to train for upcoming events. As I learn to listen to my body, I closely monitor my pain and tolerance levels. If I can continue a modified form of training while keeping an injured area below a five out of ten on my personal pain scale (where it's uncomfortable but I'm not doing further damage), then I continue with other training exercises that translate well to my sport. I hate making excuses, and I hate taking days off. Training itself is a form of therapy for me!

In the few times I've sustained a major injury, I've never broken a bone in my body (other than fracturing my nose). It's remarkable. I attribute that to a childhood full of learning how to fall. The times where I have been injured—where I couldn't move a finger or put weight on a shoulder—those were the moments when I would run to what I *did* know in my life. I would run to the Lord and say, *God, I may have screwed up Your plan for me big-time.*

If so, what do I have left? Where do we go from here? It caused me to cast my concerns on Him in a very tangible way. Whatever the crisis, the Lord is always the answer.

Injuries often come down to me making a stupid mistake or pushing myself too hard. Without the Lord protecting my heart and mind, injuries are miserable and can even lead to hopelessness. In the past, I would sometimes react with negative self-talk that would discourage me and make me afraid that I might never fully recover or be able to overcome the injury. But I love this quote from pastor and author Bill Johnson: "I can't afford to have thoughts in my head about me that God doesn't have in His." From the Bible, I confidently know how God feels about me, what His thoughts are toward me, and that nothing could ever separate me from His love.

I have to say, *Lord, my identity isn't in this, but I love this and still desire to do it well.* I'm grateful that through the injuries I've sustained I have gained a greater perspective in life. Perspective is never just what you see, but how you *view* what you see. Sometimes I've realized that the sport has had too much of a hold on my life. So I'll sit and reorganize my priorities to make sure they're in the proper God-given order.

Perseverance

One of the themes of *American Ninja Warrior* is overcoming obstacles. We have too many people who call themselves Christians who think that success is a given. That it should come overnight. We're facing a pandemic of that attitude and mentality. Our Christian walks are a process. The word "sanctification" comes to mind.

Moses was eighty years old when God called him to save His people and leave Egypt, and then the people of Israel went out into the wilderness for another forty years before they entered the Promised Land. David was a young teenager when he slew Goliath, but before he became king he set about a process of serving the current king and continually stepping out in faith. Even Jesus said there is seedtime and then harvest. Anything that's going to stand firm has to be tested. And we know that pressure creates diamonds.

I spent my entire life climbing on things and jumping on things, such that when I started training for *American Ninja Warrior*, I already had a good foundation. I got rejected two years in a row when I auditioned for the show. I thought, *God, I thought I was going to be the Kingdom Ninja. I've trained and prepared my body . . . Why is this not going the way I want?* So I joined the "walk-on line," camping out for a week outside one of the competition zones. I was tired and sunburned and dehydrated, and people in my life were telling me to give up.

And then I competed five years in a row . . . and kept falling. Every year I asked, *God, I'm giving it my all . . . why do I keep falling?* Again, not unlike life. But I discovered that the goal is to persevere and to use the platform I'm given. Every single time I'm on television, whether winning or losing or

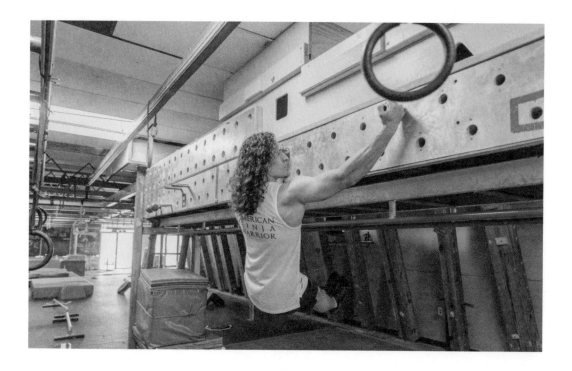

falling, I can use it as a means to promote the gospel in order to fill heaven and empty hell. That's what Christians are called to do. Over time, I felt like the Lord could trust me with more. Many millennials expect instant success, but we need to realize that it is a process, and it often takes years to reach our goals. But it's always worth it. Just don't waste your life climbing to the top of the ladder only to realize it was leaning against the wrong building. Really *know* what it is you're fighting for and chasing after in life. Will that thing truly care for you, provide for you, and satisfy? Or will it leave you wanting?

I have found my One Thing through my relationship with Christ, and three decades in, He has never left me or forsaken me. I have let myself down many times, and other people have let me down too—even friends and family. Well-intentioned Christians have let me down because they're still only human. They're not God. Don't ever trust God's people more than God, or you'll set yourself up for disappointment. But the Lord has never let me down. And the times in life when I felt like He had let me down always ended up feeling different when I gained a bit of understanding and Kingdom perspective.

My advice is to put your faith and hope and trust in Jesus Christ. The life I'm living now requires greater trust each day. God is constantly calling me to deeper places, where I feel like I'm out of my comfort zone. In Scripture, people sometimes felt like they had run out of options, yet God always stepped in and showed up and did the miraculous. Don't get angry when God puts you in positions where you're uncomfortable. Well, you *can* feel angry (it's not as if God doesn't already know how you're feeling), but regardless of the circumstances, trust Him to uphold His end of His promises in Scripture. Work to be faithful in the little things—whether it's a hobby, a social media following, or a job.

Enjoy the journey because it never ends up looking anything like what we've imagined. I'm going to keep putting one foot in front of the other, no matter what happens in my life. You can hold me to that.

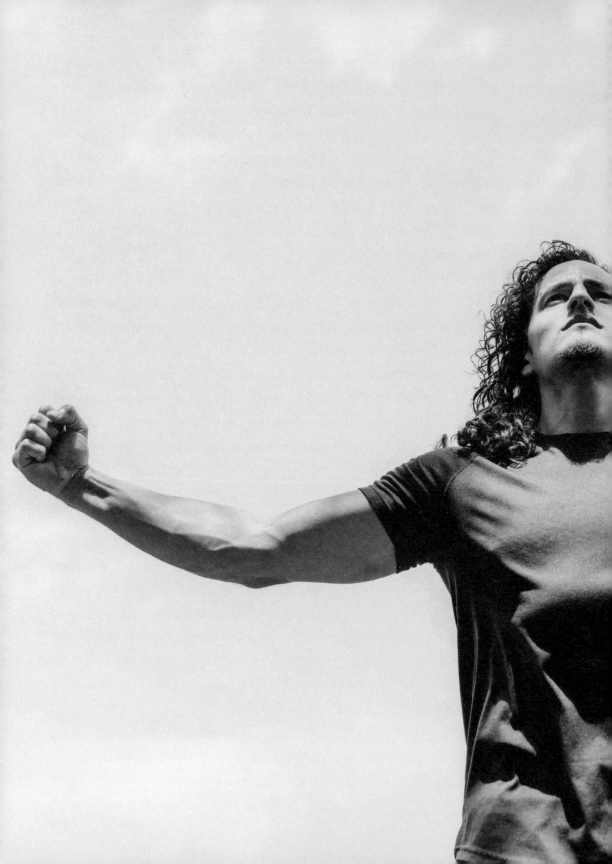

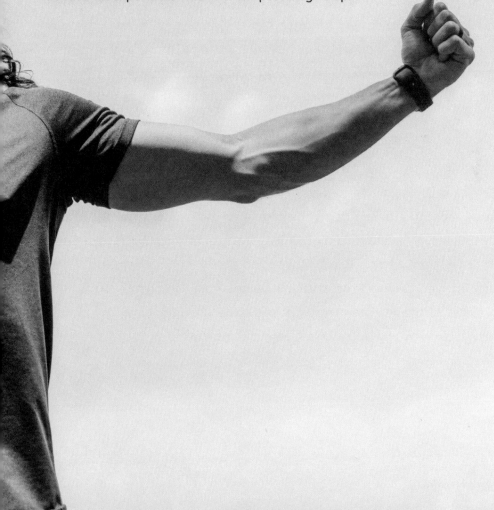

ANW SEASON 9: DOUBLE DIPPER, LAS VEGAS FINALS, STAGE 1, 2017

On the Double Dipper, you start from a very high platform, grab onto a bar, slide forward on a track (like a roller coaster), jump to another bar on another track, and dismount to the landing platform.

This was one of the only times Production ever let us practice an obstacle prior to actual competition (many of the course testers had really struggled with it). To my shock, I failed my practice attempt. I was incredibly nervous going into actual competition, but when I got there, I gave it everything I had, and to my surprise, it worked out perfectly. Then I sped through the rest of the course and finished with a great time! I often think about that experience when I'm tempted to give up.

Competition Rituals

People often ask me what my competition rituals are—whether I only eat certain foods, have lucky underwear, can't step on a crack, or things like that. Honestly, I think a lot of things like that are unnecessary and may be birthed out of fear or paranoia. Mentally, I try to stay consistent in my process, whether I'm training or competing, so that competition doesn't feel as heavy or filled with anxiety.

My only rituals are the basic physical, mental, and spiritual things I do pretty much every day. I try to get a certain number of hours of sleep the night before competition; I warm up well before leaving the hotel or place I'm staying, warm up again once I'm at the competition site, and again leading up to my run; I always wear a jacket to keep my muscles warmed and ready. I'll have a playlist of favorite hip-hop songs to drown out the noise (if there's too much around me), and once we walk through the course and watch a demonstration of success on each obstacle, I visualize the course close to a hundred times in my head (if not more) while waiting to run. I stay off my feet as much as possible if I'm running late on the list because sometimes we're there hours upon hours before running. I never put my competition shoes on until sitting on the steps on the starting line so as not to get dust or anything else on the rubber sole.

To spiritually prepare, once I'm on the platform at the starting line of any course, I always lift my hands up high, smile from ear to ear with gratitude for another opportunity to do what I love, and thank my Father God. Then I say a quick prayer, telling Him that I'll do my very best and trust Him with the results, whatever they may be this time around. I rub my hands together, yawn to relax my body, and then take off running!

DANIEL GIL: A STUDENT, FRIEND, AND COMPETITOR
BY SAM SANN

MY LIFE HAS always been a series of obstacles.

I was born in Phnom Penh, Cambodia. When I was five years old, my mother, overwhelmed with her seven children, left me and my sister to be raised by my grandmother. I will never forget her saying goodbye to me at sunset and walking away into the distance. I was so sad I cried for days. At the time I didn't understand her decision to leave me, but now I think it was destiny. If she hadn't left me with my grandmother, I may not have survived the Communist regime.

When I was nine years old, the Khmer Rouge forced everyone in my community of Battambang to leave their homes and move to the country with only what we could carry. We were forced to learn to survive in the wilderness. Shortly after, I was forced to work in the labor camps from sunup to sundown with only one meal a day. It was always the same: one cup of rice soup. I learned at a young age to become independent. I remember one night when it was raining, and I was alone and cold and did not even have a blanket. I didn't know if I would survive the night, but it never crossed my mind to give up.

When I was twelve years old, I decided to escape the labor camp and find my grandmother. I left with a friend from the camp. There was a storm and flooding, so no one noticed us leave. Unfortunately, my friend didn't make it through the flood. I finally found my grandmother's village. My grandmother told my sister and me that the Khmer Rouge was planning to exterminate the Cambodian race. We decided to leave and walked for days to the Thailand border, where we were rescued by the Red Cross. We were transported to San Diego and then Houston. Once in Houston, we stayed in YMCA housing for six months. We ended up in a poor neighborhood in Third Ward.

School was another obstacle I had to overcome. I had missed four years of school while I was in labor camps. Trying to catch up felt impossible at times. When I arrived in the United States, I did not speak any English, and I was put in classes with kids many years younger than me. I pretended to be younger so they wouldn't make fun of me for being so far behind. For many years I was bullied for my broken English and my race. I spent most of those years by myself, drawing and making sketches.

After I graduated, I worked hard and eventually started my own hair salon. I ran cross-country and track my whole life, and athletic things came easily to me. I loved rock climbing, but twelve years ago I fell and broke my knee.

After the injury I was doing rehab. The doctor informed me that I would never walk or run again. I said, "Just put me back together!" A year later I didn't know what to do to stay engaged athletically, so I built the Iron Sports gym to rehab my knee. I had been watching *Sasuke*, the Japanese version of *Ninja Warrior*. I decided to build something like that. People laughed at me and said, "You're crazy. This would make a great birthday party place." As it turned out, they hit the nail on the head. In part.

Then one day I was watching TV, and season 1 of *American Ninja Warrior* came on. Several of the top ninjas in America competed against other ninjas from around the world. The Americans were beaten badly. Being an immigrant and feeling grateful for all the opportunities this country has given me, I decided to focus my ninja warrior training gym on helping American athletes compete on the world stage. I trained many of the top ninjas who came out of Houston over the years. The gym continued to grow and became a training ground not only for adults but also for kids learning the sport.

I was the first person in the country to build a ninja gym, and there have to be upwards of 400 in the country now. The ninja movement has spread like wildfire.

If you are facing an obstacle that seems impossible, please remember: If you persevere, you can overcome anything. I'm still active in the ninja scene—still competing every year, even at age fifty-four! Daniel was my student for many years, studying under me.

When NBC found out I built a gym, they called and asked me to be on the show. That first year we had between nineteen and twenty-four competitors. Somehow, one day this curly-haired kid walks into the facility and says he wants a job. Daniel asked, "What is this place?"

"We monkey around and play and have fun," I said. "It's an obstacle course."

He came into class, and I basically tortured him and showed him a few things here and there. I taught him how to rock climb and some basics like that. My gym was known for brutal and challenging obstacles, like a Giant Peg Wheel, 51 Roulette, and a Circuit Board—all known to develop insane levels of grip, upper-body, and core strength. These are the ingredients needed by any serious ninja athlete.

A few years went by, and Daniel was getting stronger and faster. He threw himself into it full-force. I was a rock climber, so showing Daniel how to use grip and core strength was the best thing I could impart to him. He started to compete at local competitions, and when his year came in 2015, he and I actually competed together on the same course.

I enjoyed the opportunity to be on the show, but Daniel hit the scene and people were amazed. He made the course look easy! We both finished the course, but that was the only time it was ever in Houston. The entire city was rooting for us, it seemed. The next day we had an extended course—a longer and harder version of what we'd conquered the night before. Daniel had gone all the way to the Crazy Cliffhanger but fell at that spot. It was right before the end of the course. There were no finishers that entire night—right up until the time came for me to run.

"He's twice the age of most of the people he's competing against," said the announcers on the broadcast. And they pointed out that I was competing against many of the people I had trained! Thankfully, there were a lot of upper-body oriented obstacles on that course, and I consider those my specialty. So much of this sport is about strength to bodyweight ratio, and at only 138 pounds, I felt like the course played to my strengths. I hadn't cut my hair since I'd fallen on stage 1 the previous year in Las Vegas. I said I wouldn't cut it until I fell again!

I taught this kid how to do this thing, so I have to finish, I thought. With my grip strength and experience, I was the first guy in *American Ninja Warrior* history to finish the course both nights. At the end of the course I placed my hands together, sank to my knees, and hit the buzzer. I was forty-eight years old and had snapped my knee in half just a few years before.

For the next five years, Daniel didn't fall off a *Ninja Warrior* obstacle. He became a phenom in our sport and took it by storm. By season 9, he had become an independent and was trying to break a record every time he approached a course. Daniel is *very* smart. His IQ on obstacles is second to none.

I used to tell him, "It doesn't matter how strong you are; the obstacle will humble you, no matter what." His humility may be his greatest strength, and I'm very grateful for the time I had with Daniel.

I said, "Daniel, life is an obstacle. Don't fight the obstacle, like I do. You have to enjoy the obstacle and overcome it. Enjoy every obstacle, and don't fight it. Don't be like me!" He took it to another level. He kept what I taught him, and he built on it through his faith in God.

There's a new breed of ninja out there chasing Daniel. I'm training a young lady who is fourteen years old who will one day make Daniel look slow. She has a great work ethic. She has overcome things in her life.

I'm fifty-four and still competing, which, as you can imagine, comes with its share of high and low points! I went into a recent competition with a calf injury, which I didn't tell the producers about. But when I ran up the warped wall, my calf muscle popped on me. I want to be the oldest competitor on the show for as long as my body will allow. I'm not done. I'm still learning in the game, because in this game you never stop learning.

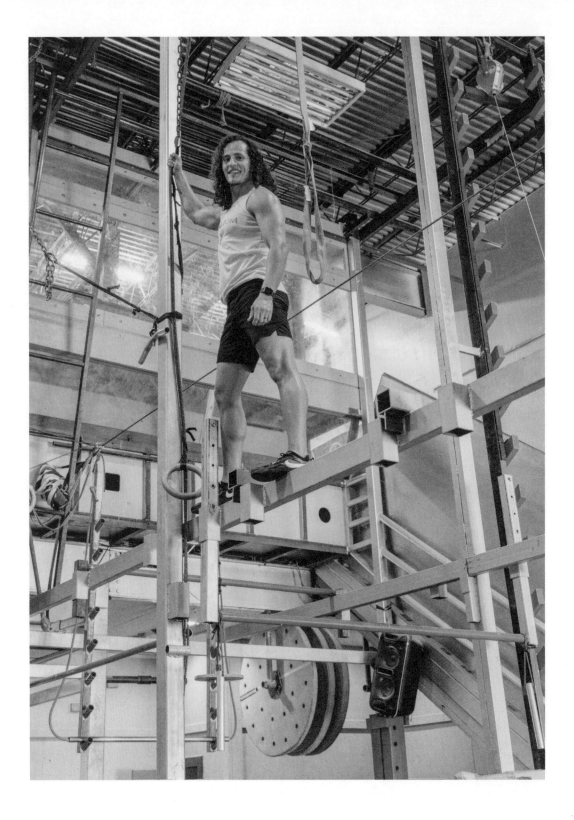

10

GIVING BACK

When I was young, I was fascinated with the idea of being on TV. Whenever I attended a church function or a sporting event where there was a guest speaker who had been on television, I was completely dialed in. The words they said would impact me more than what my coaches, teachers, or even my parents would say because "so and so" said it and "so and so" was on TV! I wanted to be like them because of the celebrity status they held and what they had achieved.

Eventually, as I matured a bit, I began to realize that not all celebrities have it together, and many really aren't great role models for children. So when I started to compete on television, I realized I would have the same kind of impact on young people that others had on me. But I wanted to tell them the things that I needed to hear at their age, the things that I want a celebrity to tell *my* future kids—because I was having an impact on somebody's kid, potentially influencing their future! (No pressure.) What did I want them to remember about me? What did I want them to take away from the conversation or experience and remember the next time they saw me compete?

Primarily, through the show, I wanted to point people to the Kingdom of God (hence the whole "Kingdom Ninja" thing). But also to let them know that they are capable of overcoming *any* obstacles they'll face in life. I want them to know that hard work truly does pay off, and no matter how many times you fall or fail, you learn to get back up as quickly as possible so you can finish what you started. And never forget to encourage, inspire, and motivate people along the way as much as you can because we *all* have people looking at our lives and watching how we live them. Everyone carries a level of influence. You might not have millions of followers or thousands of subscribers or be featured in media as a big shot, but we all have families, friends, and peers who take note of our lives and how we handle their many hurdles. What we do with our words and actions truly does affect others, for better or for worse.

It took me by surprise when people started to recognize me as a celebrity at the mall or my grocery store, take photos, ask for an autograph, or tell me how much their kids (or grandma) adored me! Still, it was something I had dreamed about for a long time when I was training and preparing for the show, even when I had no guarantee of it ever actually working out. *American Ninja Warrior* would have zero place in my life if I wasn't chasing with all my heart after the Lord. At the end of the day, whenever I'm showcased or featured on this very curated show, I want the segment to be encouraging, inspirational, and pointing in the direction of the Lord. Growing up in a Christian household, and now with my wife, I've had people to check me. There is an artifice that can come from being on television and having a little fame. Anytime my head begins to swell, it's immediately popped by my sweet Abby. The mentors and leaders in my life provide a sounding board as well. There is wisdom in counsel.

I have access to more people now when I need help. I have my wife and family but also a network of people that I can get wisdom from. My dear friend, Randy Caldwell, once told me, "There are two ways of learning in life—from my mistakes or from your own." So I learn as much as I can from

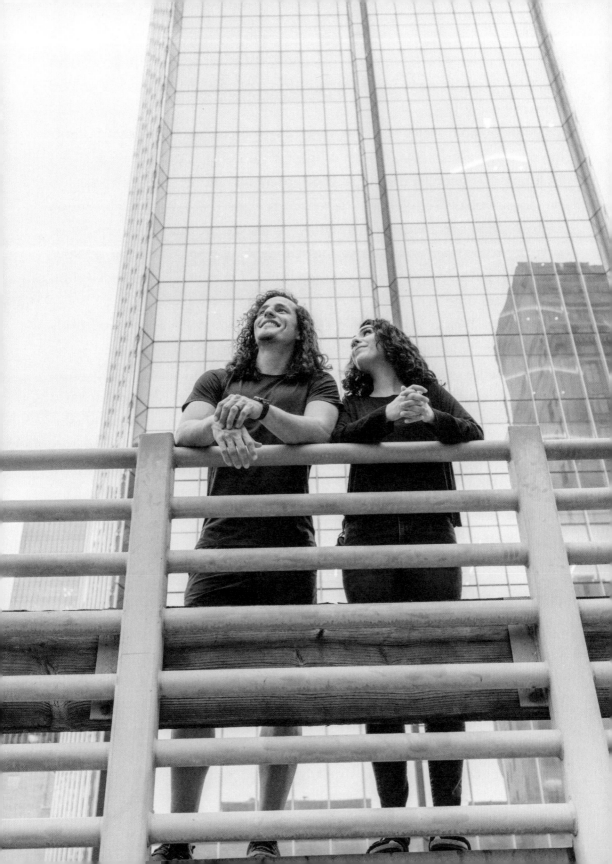

him and others who have taken me under their wings over the years. This has been an extra benefit of whatever fame or celebrity status I've gained from the show.

Oddly, being on television or writing a book often has the effect of granting a person perspective. Fame, at least in America, is as relative or siloed as it has ever been, in the sense that entertainment content continues to be segmented and audience-directed. Back when there were four television networks and cable was in its infancy, it meant a lot more to be on television, because there was a sense that the whole nation would see it. Now, with so many streaming services, more people are showcased on TV than at any other time in history!

All of which is to say, I have a sense that the show's reach is relatively small, and my window on the show itself is going to be relatively short in the grand scheme of things. So in light of that, what am I doing to maximize every moment and opportunity? I understand that *Ninja Warrior* reaches a niche audience, but even so, I want to try to demonstrate a healthy relationship with fame. I don't want to need it, and I don't want to chase it as if it were an idol in my life. As my mentor said, I can learn from my mistakes or from someone else's! Some have to touch the flame to understand it's a bad idea, but I'll try to avoid as many unnecessary pitfalls as I can by learning from others.

Being a Role Model

I cannot begin to tell you the number of messages I have received over the years about being a role model to kids and even adults who have watched me compete over the seasons. It is truly the most humbling thing about the show and a joy that I experience regularly! Online messages are often hard to respond to quickly because I try to do it myself, and I hate how impersonal social media feels. But when I meet people in real life in a store, traveling, or walking down the street, it brings a joy that few other things in

OVERCOMING LABELS: THE OPERA NINJA

My first year on *American Ninja Warrior*, I told the producers about my background as a classical vocalist, multi-year All-State choir member, competitive solo and ensemble performer, and worship leader at my local church. I have also performed with organizations in Houston that produce operas, classical concerts, musicals and plays, and other performance art.

Ninja Warrior really zoned in on the opera schtick and wanted to label me the Opera Ninja! Thankfully, I didn't let it stick and instead became known for the Kingdom, because I wanted the show to be a ministry for me. But *still*, people often ask me if I'm the Opera Ninja! You may get labeled something in life that you're not a fan of, but what's most important is, Did you answer to it? Or did you correct them?

life do. After being recognized and excitedly asked if I'm "that guy from the ninja show," or most of the time very specifically if I'm "Daniel Gil the Kingdom Ninja," I then have the opportunity to make someone's day or even a memory that they will never ever forget. And I say that because I pretty clearly remember every time in life when I met a celebrity somewhere and how cool (or sometimes terrible) it was! I've heard horror stories of when people met celebrities and were sorely disappointed in their better-than-you attitude. I'm not anywhere near the level of Hollywood's superstars, but I do get recognized often, and I truly desire that every interaction with a fan is a great interaction.

I've put that same mentality toward my coaching. I've now been coaching ninja for around ten years, and it's truly humbling to see the impact I've had on former students. Over the past couple of years, I've had people come up to me and thank me for being a coach to them when they were younger. For always taking care of them and being a great coach. For celebrating them and how they grew stronger over time. And now they're graduating from college and moving forward in life.

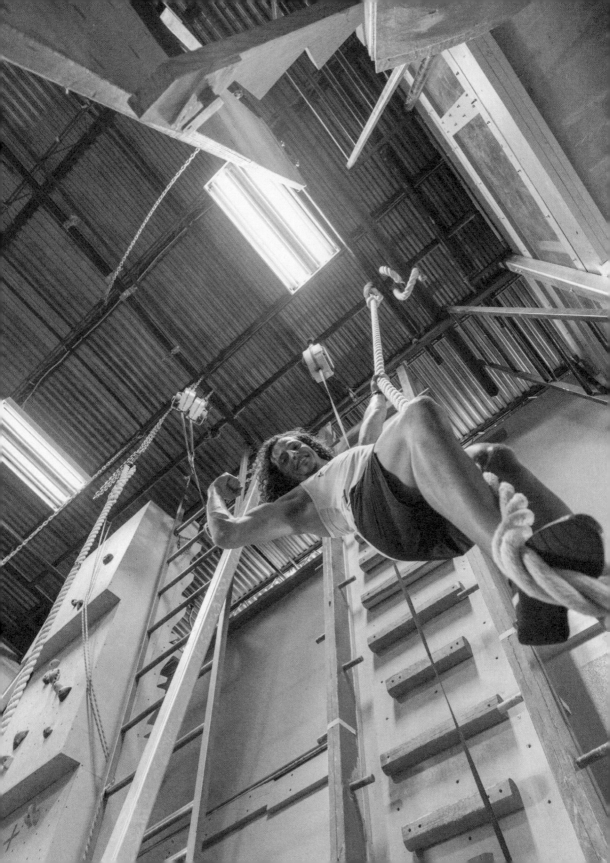

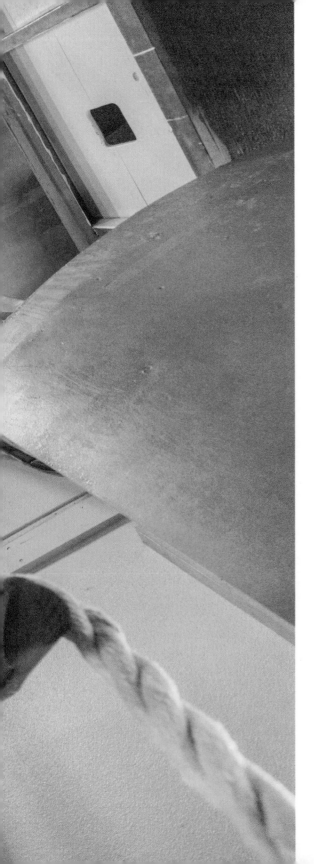

Thrill Seeking, Risk, and Manhood

I love reading. I've read a lot of books about being a strong, independent man of God. Woven into our DNA as men is finding what our limitations are and pushing those limitations. As a kid, I wanted to ride the biggest, fastest, most extreme roller coasters because I wanted to say I'd tamed them!

Many men don't consciously recognize that need, but they pursue those appetites in destructive ways. We need to push those envelopes in healthy ways because that desire is woven into every man. Even Jesus didn't rebuke the disciples when they were arguing over who was the greatest. He simply redefined greatness as serving others.

For me, I have a desire to teach the Word of God to others and find out how much I can learn, grow, and understand. As an athlete, I want to get as much information as I can so I can build the best training routines and stretch myself to the limit in these competitions. There will always be opportunities to have the thrill of adventure and push yourself to the limits, to see what you're made of. You might not think you're much of anything right now, but I promise you, you can be.

To the Parents of Young Athletes

Many kids are joining ninja gyms with dreams of making it onto the main show or the junior circuit. With these dreams, there comes a lot of investment from parents and lots of expectations. Parents, you need to really *know* your child and understand their goals, while at the same time encouraging them to learn and grow. It's finding that balance of stretching them out of their comfort zone while at the same time keeping the perspective of *why* they're doing it.

I see parents wanting their kids to do well *way* more than their child does (not that the child doesn't also want to do well). It leads to kids feeling, *On the good days, Mom and Dad love me, and I feel great. But on the bad days, they're disappointed in me, and I feel terrible.* The best thing is to have a healthy enough relationship with your kids to be able to challenge and encourage them without exasperating them or robbing the joy from their sport or activity. That kind of relationship takes time and intentionality.

In the gym, some of my students will fall and immediately look at their mom and dad to see what their reaction will be . . . in fear that the reaction will be one of anger or disappointment. Some look around to see if *anyone* is there watching. *Someone* needs to care! If the mom and dad aren't around, the responsibility defaults to me—the coach—and I do the best I can to speak life and encouragement over that child the few hours a week I see them.

The best parents will tell their kids how proud they are because even *attempting* an obstacle can be difficult at times. They're supportive in a way that's unique to their child. Effective parents are intentional enough to know *how* to communicate with their children.

I'm forever grateful for my mom, who recognized my strengths in life as a kid and always encouraged me to steward them well—in sports and otherwise. She not only prioritized educating me and my siblings with homeschooling but also noted each of our unique gifts and talents. She's always been a good sounding board for us and always wanted to see her children succeed. She was the *loudest*, most excited parent at every single sporting game I ever played! Regardless of the outcome, she championed us and helped us to learn and grow. That's the kind of support your kid needs and what will help them thrive.

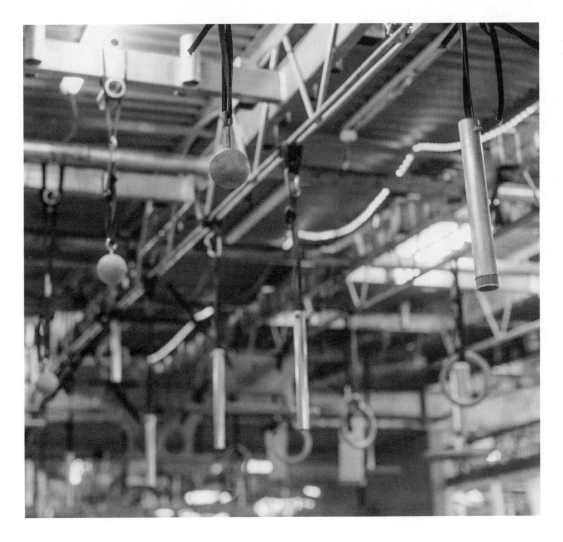

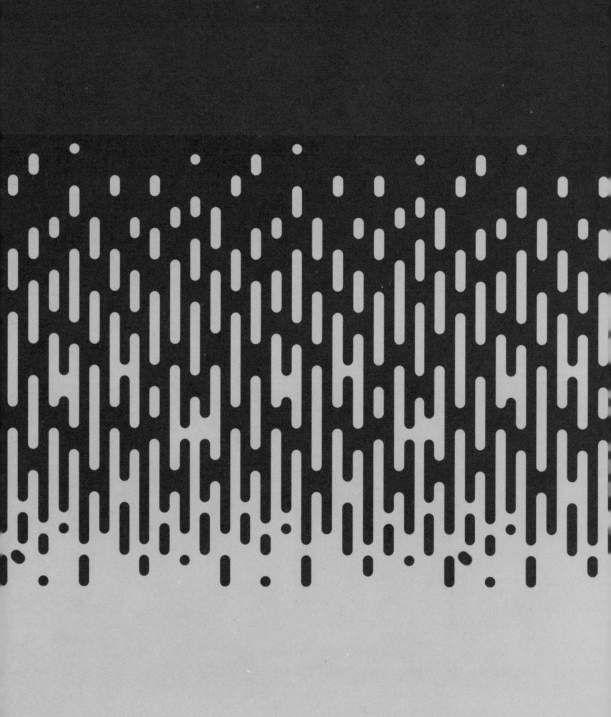

PART
THREE

SPIRITUAL
HEALTH

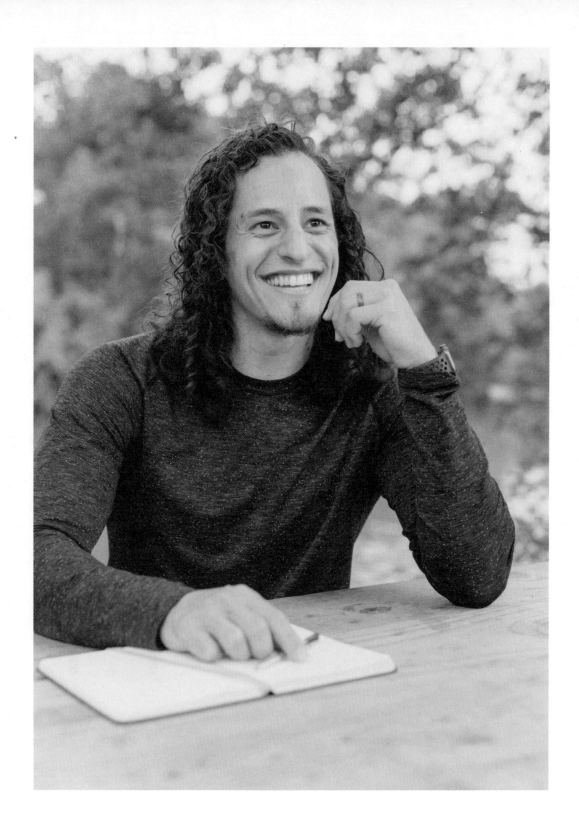

11

A LIFE
OF FAITH

The final part of this book is the most important: Spiritual Health. I believe we are not just bodies and minds but also souls. If our bodies are fit and our minds are steady but our souls are not right, then we are missing something crucial about our lives and what it means to be human.

I was born, raised, and homeschooled right in my hometown of Houston, Texas. I was one of five siblings. I'm the second oldest, and while I was growing up I was pretty much involved in every church-based organization you can imagine. I owe my spiritual walk to my parents and my church, who invested in me as a kid and taught me the Word of God. Like the Bible says, I was planted by streams of water (Psalm 1:3). I was involved in everything from Kingdom Clowns ministry (this is a real thing) to Kingdom Mimes ministry (yep, this too), sign language ministry, nursing home ministry, and more. I was probably *doing* a lot of Christian things long before I even really understood what it truly meant to *be* a Christian. But I definitely grew a deep love for people during that season of my life, and that has stayed with me to this day. When I was younger, I was a very shy kid in public. At first, I was really uncomfortable visiting nursing homes, homeless shelters, and places for adults with developmental disabilities because they were different from me, and that scared me at first. Over time, the Lord began to give me a heart for other people as I saw just how much impact it had when I offered a genuine smile, a listening ear, a word of encouragement, or a basic necessity to someone in need. I saw their eyes light up when they realized a group had come to visit them in their distress or loneliness to provide love, support, comfort, and hope.

My mom once prayed a prayer out of desperation that went something like this: "Lord, I don't know what to do. I have all of these kids . . . God, if You'll take care of these kids . . . they need Your covering and Your guidance. I'll do my part if You'll do Yours." And the Lord was faithful.

I was about seven or eight years old when I made a commitment to Christ, making Him the Lord and leader of my life. Like a lot of us who grew up in Christian environments, I prayed a salvation prayer, indicating that I knew that Christ had died on the cross for my sins and that I wanted to go to heaven and not hell. I knew and understood the fact that I was a sinner, that I did bad things (often intentionally), and that I needed to repent and make Him the Lord and leader of my life.

In high school I really started to experience and understand that the world is truly "anti-Christ." I started feeling pressure from friends, peers, TV, movies, and music to act a certain way, talk a certain way, and *be* a certain way. I was trying on a certain amount of "worldliness" (or at least thinking about trying it on) in the way that a lot of homeschool kids (who feel uncool) often do. I remember praying a life-changing prayer when I was fourteen or fifteen: *Lord, I know I'm a Christian, but I have so many external temptations and pressures, and I'm making a lot of mistakes. If I'm going to call myself a Christian—a Christ follower—I need to really, fully give You my life, including everything that makes me, me—the good, the bad, the ugly, as well as all my fears and doubts, hopes and dreams.* Things truly changed for me from that moment onward.

I went from being someone who loved the Lord in a conceptual way because of my upbringing, to someone who was completely *sold out* to

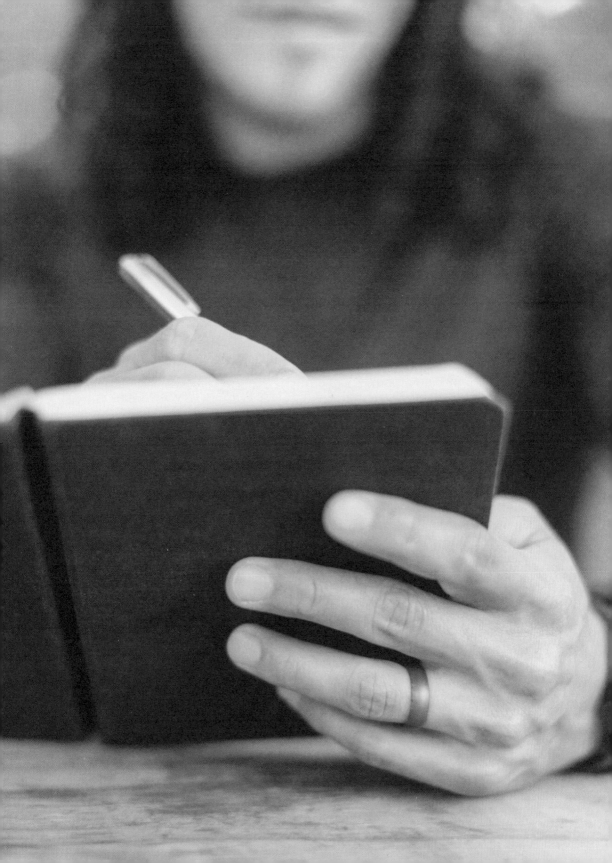

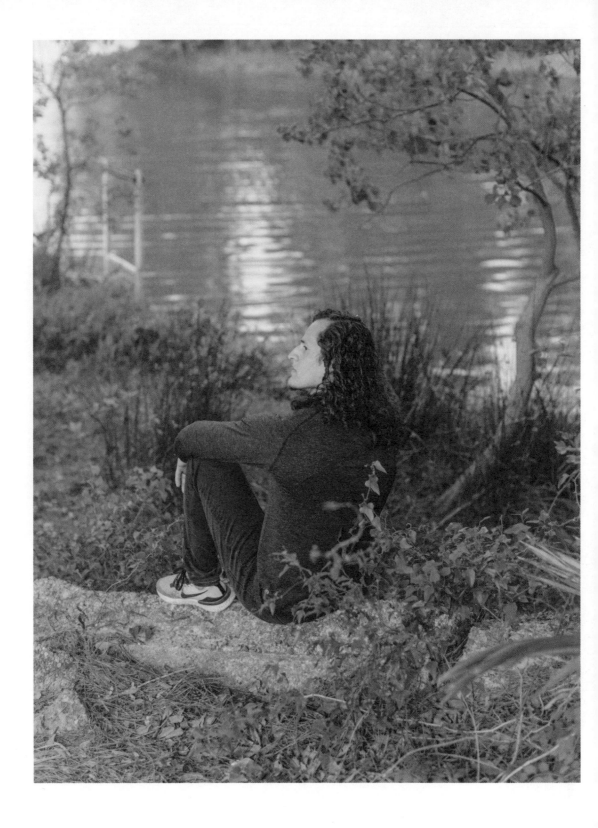

pursuing my relationship with the Lord. I took ownership of my faith. I chose not to live off my parents' faith or my pastors' faith, but to fully step into my own journey of walking with the Lord. Every relationship is a two-way street, and I began actively participating on my end to really know this God that I believe in. I read my Bible every day to better understand who He is and what He's like, to discover His character and nature, and to find my place and purpose in His beautiful design. I'm still blown away daily by what I find in the Word. I also got more connected in my church and started volunteering there as a greeter, which eventually grew to leadership roles and even becoming a worship leader by playing bass in the band and singing. As I put my life in God's hands and began to use all my gifts and talents and abilities for Him and for His glory, I saw Him honor that. I got opportunities to share the gospel that there is a God, He is good, and Jesus is the only way.

Only in Christianity does God not say, "Be good enough, and maybe I'll let you into heaven." Instead, God chooses to say, "I know you're not good enough. I know you never will be. But I love you so much that I'll show you what real, perfect love looks like and provide everything you need to know Me and walk with Me now and receive heaven in the future. In your life this love will look like sacrifice, repentance, and forgiveness."

In high school, I didn't know if I would go into business of some kind or become a singer, dancer, actor, or performer. I didn't know if I would go into ministry full-time as a pastor, worship director, or overseas missionary—all of those were huge parts of my life that I enjoyed doing already. But I decided to go to a Bible school for two years, where I could learn practical ways to share the gospel with people and to let my light shine before men (Matthew 5:16).

I wanted people to look at my life and ask, "Something is different about you—what is it?" I got to travel to places like Bulgaria, Italy, Japan, Malaysia, and Honduras, speaking, singing, and leading worship. I got to see signs, wonders, and miracles—just like I had read about in the Bible. The Bible came alive to me in ways I had only read about, and it truly changed

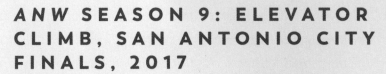

ANW SEASON 9: ELEVATOR CLIMB, SAN ANTONIO CITY FINALS, 2017

Elevator Climb was the tenth and final obstacle of the city finals courses that season. Hanging from independent handle bars, you crank each side up to ascend forty feet to the finish platform, where the buzzer is.

I was the last runner of the night, and nobody else had finished the course. It was all on me, and I was feeling the pressure like never before! But right before I stepped up to the starting line, I received encouragement from the first man to ever summit Mount Midoriyama, Geoff Britten. His voice rang in my ears throughout my run and helped give me the strength to complete the Elevator Climb. While climbing, I closed my eyes and prayed to finish this obstacle even though my arms and hands burned like never before. I became the only finisher of the San Antonio Finals course!

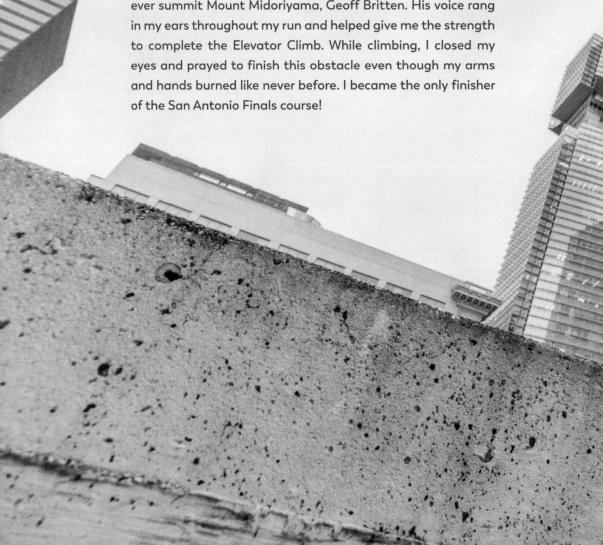

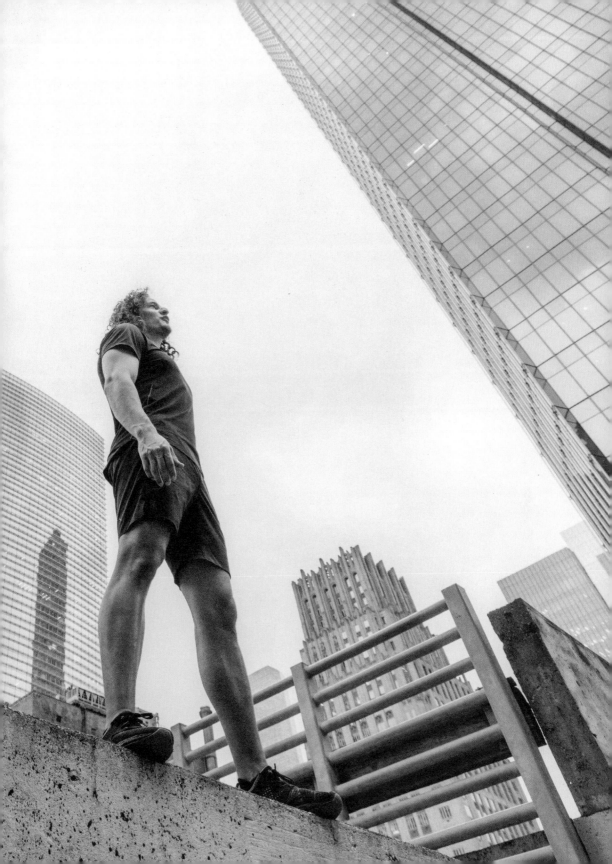

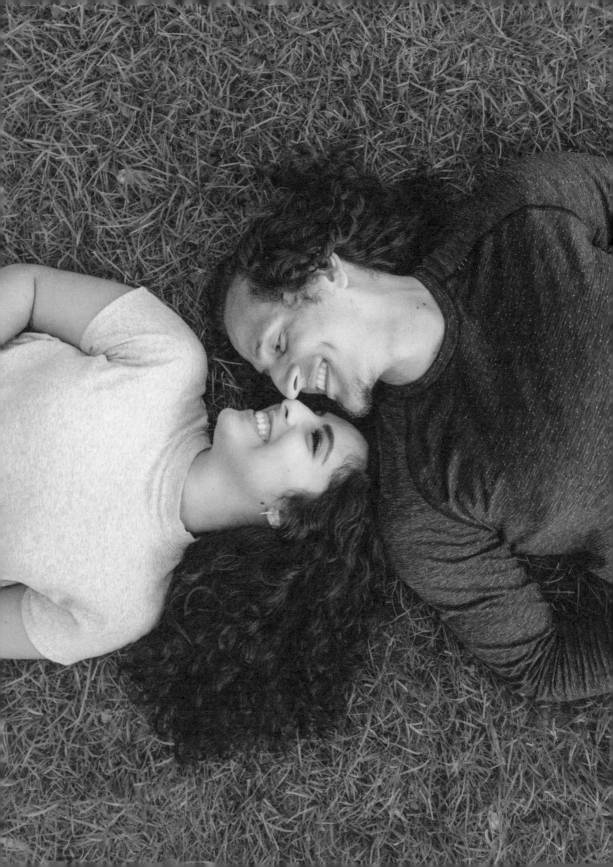

almost everything about my life. I've discovered that walking with the Lord is the most gratifying, satisfying, and fulfilling life there is even on difficult days. It is the reason I was born: to know and be known by God. My faith came to life in all kinds of new ways during those two foundational years at Bible school.

At about that time, a friend let me know that there was a job open in a ninja gym. I thought, *Lord if You're going to open a door for me to do these ninja competitions, I want to use my gifts, talents, and abilities to spread the gospel in that area.* That's how the Kingdom Ninja concept came to be.

I'm trying to put *everything* in my life into His hands, knowing that He is good and has a plan (or many) to get me where He wants me to be so I can do what He asks me to do. It's a daily walk of faith.

> *In the same way, let your light shine before others, so that they may see your good works and give glory to your Father who is in heaven.*
>
> MATTHEW 5:16

Joyfulness

Joyfulness is a big part of my life. It's a key identifier to others that is showcased in everything I do, whether leading worship, speaking to groups, or competing on *American Ninja Warrior*. Joy truly radiates through every aspect of my life. And it's not something I fabricate or have any control over. My joy is based solely in my relationship with God. You see, the Christian idea of joyfulness is different from happiness because happiness can change.

Happiness is circumstantial; it comes and goes by the day. But the joy of my salvation as a believer in Christ is constant and ever-present regardless of what may be going on in my life. The fear, anxiety, pain, loss, and regrets that God has redeemed in my life have literally transformed me from the inside out during my time walking with Him. Thankfulness is tied to my joy because I know I have been saved, delivered, and set free from the curse of separation from God.

There is truly so much joy available and freely given to us when we walk with Christ and live for Him. Specifically, 1 Peter 1:8 refers to a joy that is unspeakable and full of gladness. The Bible says that Jesus had more joy than all His companions (Hebrews 1:9, quoting Psalm 45:7) and that "the joy of the LORD is your strength" (Nehemiah 8:10). The Bible also says joy is a fruit of the Spirit (Galatians 5:22), which means that if I'm walking with God, then joy should grow and become evident in my life for others to see. Joy isn't a personality trait but is instead one of the greatest gifts of God— so valuable that the Bible says Jesus suffered the cross, enduring its shame, all for the joy that was set before Him (Hebrews 12:2).

That's not to say I never go through tough times, pain, and grief, or that I never make regrettable mistakes. On this side of heaven, trouble will always be possible. But what I am saying is that I have a limitless source of joy because of Jesus, and nothing else in this life comes anywhere close to that joy. If you've ever wondered about my joy, well, now you know where it comes from and what it means to me.

Spiritual Disciplines

I'm very practical when it comes to spiritual growth and maturity. The level of discipline that I put toward training, speaking, or singing is the same level of discipline I put toward my walk with the Lord. I never wanted to say a prayer just as a "get out of hell free" card. I truly want to know the Lord and what He's like. I also truly believe that is possible in this life. I continually pursue Him and fellowship with Him.

The New Testament letter of 1 John says that staying in fellowship with the Lord helps make our joy complete. I study Scripture and look at the stories of men and women who made mistakes and were imperfect but continued to act in faith to do what the Lord had called them to. (Of course, some didn't follow God or act in faith, but we can learn from that too.)

Gideon had very poor "self-talk," and God had to change it (Judges 6:15).

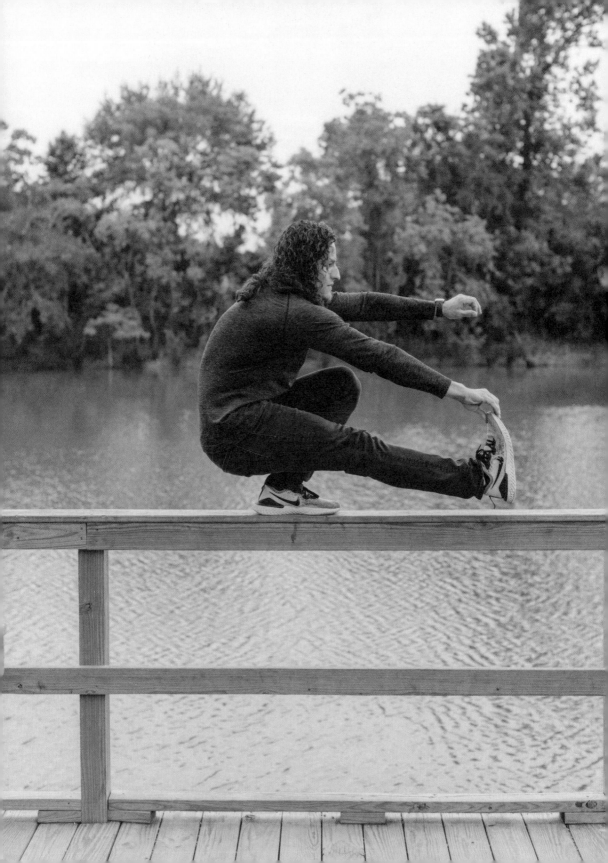

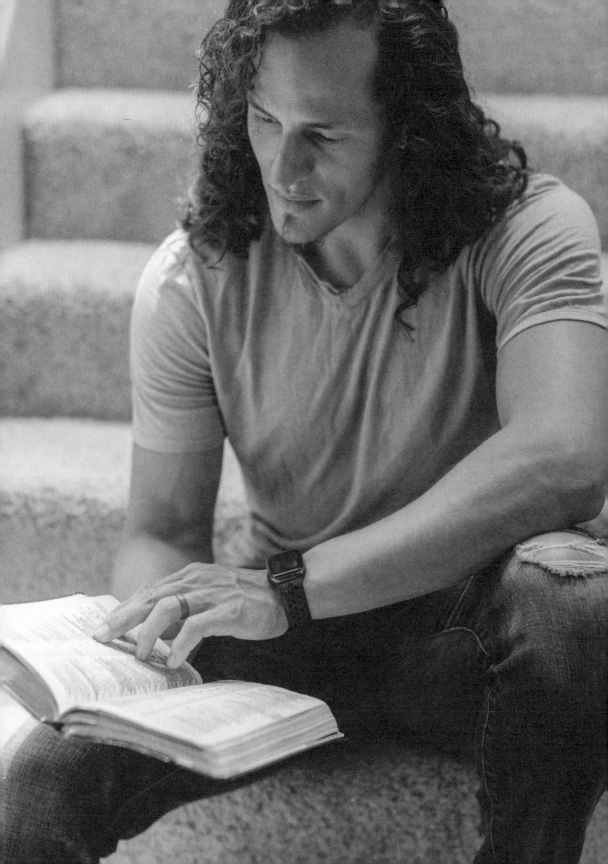

Moses didn't think he could communicate effectively, so God had to use Moses's brother, Aaron, while He built Moses's confidence (Exodus 4:10-16). Peter talked so much that he put his foot in his mouth, and Jesus had to humble him by revealing his flawed perspective (Matthew 16:22-23).

In addition to the Bible, I also love reading spiritual biographies. There's a series called God's Generals that talks about different men and women throughout history who have stewarded revivals. Another book, *Dreaming with God* by pastor Bill Johnson, transformed the way that I envision my life, limitations, and future endeavors with the Lord and what He can do with my life.

Reading the Bible and Prayer

Bible reading and prayer doesn't have to be complicated. Start with day one, right where you are, and with what you have. Start by setting realistic goals, like reading a chapter of the Bible a day, or even meditating on a single verse throughout the day. A dear friend of mine, Randy Caldwell, explained it to me like this: "Information leads to knowledge; knowledge leads to understanding; understanding builds your trust; and trust releases your faith." You get that through reading the Word of God, and I've never read the Bible the same way since. Another influencer I really connect with is Ruslan Karaoglanov (@RuslanKD), and I've heard him say we need to know which parts of the Word are *descriptive* and which are *prescriptive*. Is what you're reading simply stating what happened (for better or for worse), or is something deeper being prescribed as the God-given method of living?

We know that the Word is living and active and can change our hearts. So meditating on that day's verse or chapter throughout the day will literally change our hearts and our actions from the inside out. It's a miraculous thing. Whatever we fill ourselves up with, that is what will come out of us in life. When the world puts pressure on me, I want the Word of God to come out of me, because I truly believe that the answer to every question we could ever have in life can ultimately be found in the Word of God. Often, people just don't look that hard.

One example of this was when I first found out about the ninja gym and was over the moon about the possibility of working there, only to have the owner say, "Thanks but no thanks, and can I interest you in buying a membership?" As I left the gym, I prayed to God in my frustration and sadness and reaffirmed my trust in Him. I put it in His hands. I still needed a job and still wanted to compete on *Ninja Warrior*. But I wouldn't let my circumstances dictate my walk or faith in God no matter how frustrated I was.

Here's another example. When I competed on the show after being rejected two years in a row, I didn't hide anything from God. Even in emotional moments like that, I want to be speaking to Him and trusting Him with the results and outcomes. I know that I have value and worth in His eyes regardless of any athletic achievement I could ever attain.

The past four years have been extremely trying and difficult to understand, even as a believer. For season 11, I finally made it to the end and attempted stage 4—only to lose a million dollars by mere seconds. The next year, in season 12, I came back and won . . . but during the height of the pandemic there was no million-dollar grand prize, and I walked away with a tenth of what I could have won. The next year, in season 13, I had my eyes on the prize but then caught COVID two days before flying out to the finals.

And then for season 14, there was a requirement for all athletes to be fully vaccinated. Instead of competing, I chose to focus my attention on many projects that had been on the back burner. People were calling and saying, "You must be so devastated!" Well, if *Ninja Warrior* were my entire life, I would be devastated. But it's not—it's just a season of my life. Yes, it's currently a large part of my life, but it's not where I find my eternal value or worth. My worth is not in being on TV or competing.

When faced with the decision to compete or not, I took it to the Lord and asked Him what I should do. Now personally, I'm a guy who doesn't put *anything*—even pain meds or an allergy pill—into my body if I don't

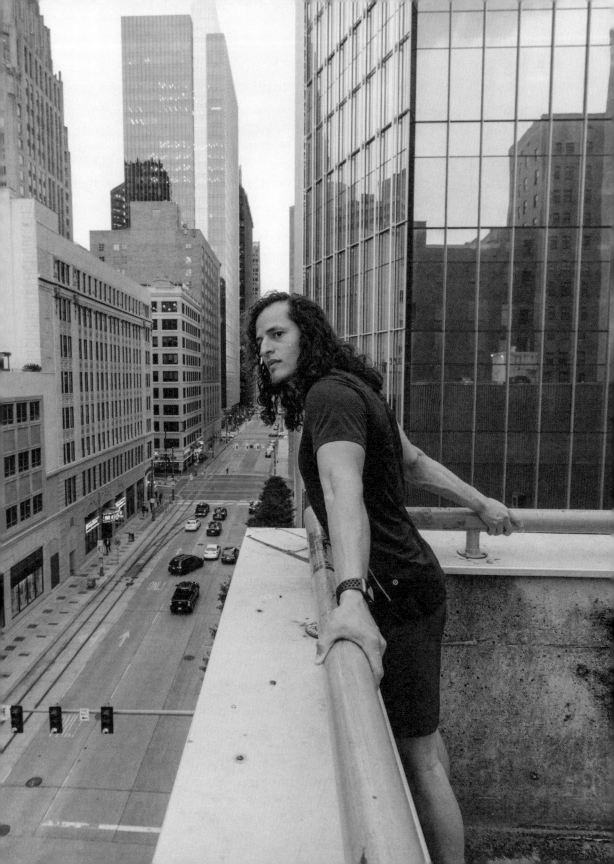

absolutely have to. I'm all for medical science, but after getting sick and making a fast, full recovery the year before, I had no desire to get a vaccine. (I'm not downplaying the effects or the severity of the virus on some people. Only the effects and severity that the virus had on me personally.) I was still open to the Lord leading me to get vaccinated if it would serve a greater good, and I didn't want whatever I decided to be seen as any kind of political statement. I sought counsel from wise people on both ends of the spectrum, prayed about it for months, and did my best to research and study on my own. But ultimately, I decided not to get the vaccine, and with no allowance for religious or medical exemptions, I chose not to compete in 2022.

I am disappointed, and I *do* wish things were different, but I also believe that every decision in life must be made in faith, understanding that God knows our hearts and that He is a rewarder of those who diligently seek Him (Hebrews 11:6). I believe that every time one door closes, another one opens up (or we finally turn and see it was open already). I'm not one to dwell on the past either. We live and learn, trust and obey, and keep putting one foot in front of the other. It's not called walking by faith for nothing.

I believe that Scripture is perfect and is given for my benefit and betterment. I'm a big fan of daily steps—even if they're small, as long as they're bringing continued growth. A daily devotional time with the Lord, listening to worship music or a podcast in your car as you drive, reading a chapter of Proverbs a day, taking notes to messages you hear and going over them later, journaling and meditating, and having biblical conversations with friends and leaders—those are things I do regularly to feed myself spiritually. The goal of my daily life is to feed my spirit more than I feed my flesh. Those two parts of me will be in conflict for the rest of my life.

I'm not perfect, and I still have to work through my own problems that I cause or sometimes simply find myself in. But everything that I'm doing, I'm trying to do as unto the Lord.

I always keep my phone close because I store my notebooks online, and

I jot down my thoughts, ideas, prayers, gratitude, and revelations as God brings them to my attention each day. I want to cultivate a spirit of thankfulness and be able to talk about the things of the Lord and share them at a moment's notice.

Life Verses

Since the Bible is such a crucial part of who I am, here are several verses that have really impacted my life.

> *One of the teachers of the law came and heard them debating. Noticing that Jesus had given them a good answer, he asked him, "Of all the commandments, which is the most important?" "The most important one," answered Jesus, "is this: 'Hear, O Israel: The Lord our God, the Lord is one. Love the Lord your God with all your heart and with all your soul and with all your mind and with all your strength.' The second is this: 'Love your neighbor as yourself.' There is no commandment greater than these."*
>
> MARK 12:28-31 NIV

As a believer, my number one priority in life is my relationship with the Lord. My heart, soul, mind, and strength are given to know Him and walk in close fellowship with Him. If that gets neglected, then everything else will be affected. All other relationships come second to Him because out of my love for Him I love people better, the way I should.

> *Let love and faithfulness never leave you; bind them around your neck, write them on the tablet of your heart. Then you will win favor and a good name in the sight of God and man. Trust in the LORD with all your heart and lean not on your own understanding; in all your ways submit to him, and he will make your paths straight .*
>
> PROVERBS 3:3-6 NIV

An attitude of love and faithfulness speaks volumes to God and to people.

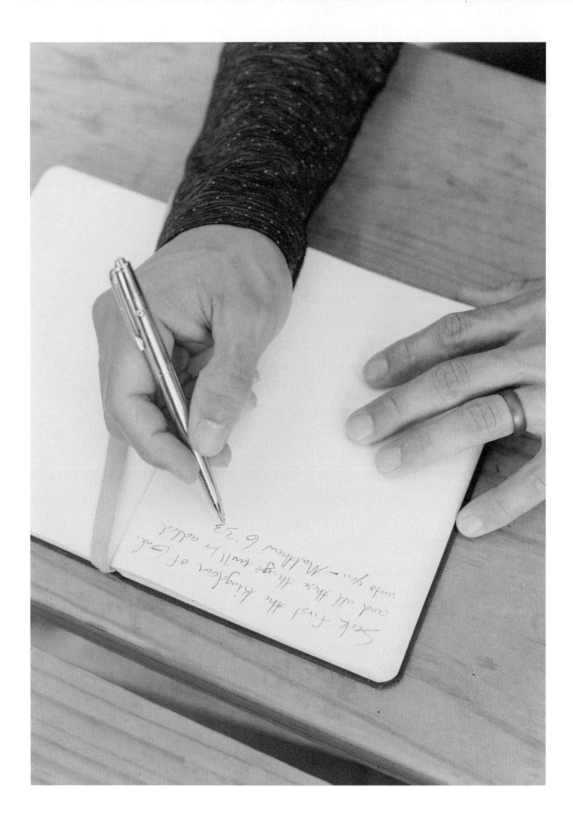

A consistent lifestyle speaks even louder and brings favor from God and people. Trusting the Lord with everything I am, even when I don't understand, and submitting to His leadership in what I do and where I go means that even in the highs and lows of life, I know He is with me and directing my path.

Do not worry, saying, "What shall we eat?" or "What shall we drink?" or "What shall we wear?" For after all these things the Gentiles seek. For your heavenly Father knows that you need all these things. But seek first the kingdom of God and His righteousness, and all these things shall be added to you. Therefore do not worry about tomorrow, for tomorrow will worry about its own things. Sufficient for the day is its own trouble .

MATTHEW 6:31-34 NKJV

The Lord knows our needs and loves us more than we know, so as a believer, I don't have to waste my time, energy, and creative thoughts by worrying about my provision. My focus and priority are set on His Kingdom and living rightly before Him, knowing and trusting that He will meet my needs. I have future plans, but I take life and its worries one day at a time.

Delight yourself also in the LORD, and He shall give you the desires of your heart. . . . The steps of a good man are ordered by the LORD, and He delights in his way. Though he fall, he shall not be utterly cast down; For the LORD upholds him with His hand.

PSALM 37:4, 23-24

The longer I walk with God, the more exciting life gets! As I have made the Lord my delight over the years, He has fulfilled dreams that were already in my heart and given me new dreams that I get to walk out with Him. I can trust that He's ordering my steps as I take them with Him, and when I fall in life, He upholds me and lifts me back up even if others give up on me.

The man who finds a wife finds a treasure, and he receives favor from the LORD.

PROVERBS 18:22 NLT

I think about this verse daily and am always full of gratitude and joy for my beautiful wife, Abigail. The Lord gave her to me for purpose and pleasure, and with each year she becomes more of a treasure to me as we pursue Him together.

We know that all things work together for good to those who love God, to those who are the called according to His purpose.

ROMANS 8:28 NKJV

Love God. Trust Him. Remember that you are called and that He has plans and purposes for you. Your situation will work out for good, even when it doesn't look or feel like it. Have faith and watch Him be faithful to His Word.

David, after he had served the purpose of God in his own generation, fell asleep and was buried among his fathers and experienced decay [in the grave].

ACTS 13:36 AMP

Other than Jesus, King David is my favorite example of someone who walked faithfully with God all his life and was a man after His own heart. Like David, I want to serve and fulfill the purposes of God in my life and for my generation before I pass on or Christ returns.

Joyful are people of integrity, who follow the instructions of the LORD. Joyful are those who obey his laws and search for him with all their hearts. They do not compromise with evil, and they walk only in his paths. You have charged us to keep your commandments carefully. Oh, that my actions would consistently reflect your decrees! Then I will not be ashamed when I compare my life with your commands. As I learn your righteous regulations, I will thank you by living as I should!

PSALM 119:1-7 NLT

This passage is essentially my own heartfelt cry to the Lord over the years, and it resonates with me strongly. I value character, integrity, intentionality, active pursuit, and daily progression toward His best for my life and the lives of those I affect. I try to learn and grow each day through reading Scripture. Every command in Scripture is there for our protection and offers many benefits for this life. Are we perfect? Never. Can we get closer each day? Absolutely.

Dreaming Big

What does it mean to dream big?

Well, practically speaking, I believe that it has to do with imagining how your calling (what you feel destined to do) and your vocation (your job or career that's currently paying the bills) may collide. When you ask yourself, *Where do my desires for the Kingdom of God line up with where God is leading me? What could that look like?*—that's dreaming big.

Often we miss out on incredible opportunities because we think too small. I've been guilty of that many times or have even disqualified myself before taking half a step on a new path before me. We believe too little in both God and ourselves. We don't trust, and we barely have any hope. But we need hope because hope breeds faith. And without faith, you won't act on your God-given goals and dreams. Hope is the confident expectation of the goodness of God in any scenario. That is the foundation that my faith is built on. I'm only speaking from my personal experience as someone who has achieved many dreams in my life already.

I've been blessed to do global missions work, travel for a living, win *Ninja Warrior*, marry the woman of my dreams, be self-employed, witness miracles with my own eyes, and enjoy countless other things that may not mean anything to you but have meant everything to me. The takeaway is to ponder your future—not selfishly thinking, *What do I want?* but instead, *What do I have, and how can I use it?* And then using every gift and talent within your control for good. Start to daydream about it and watch how God begins to move.

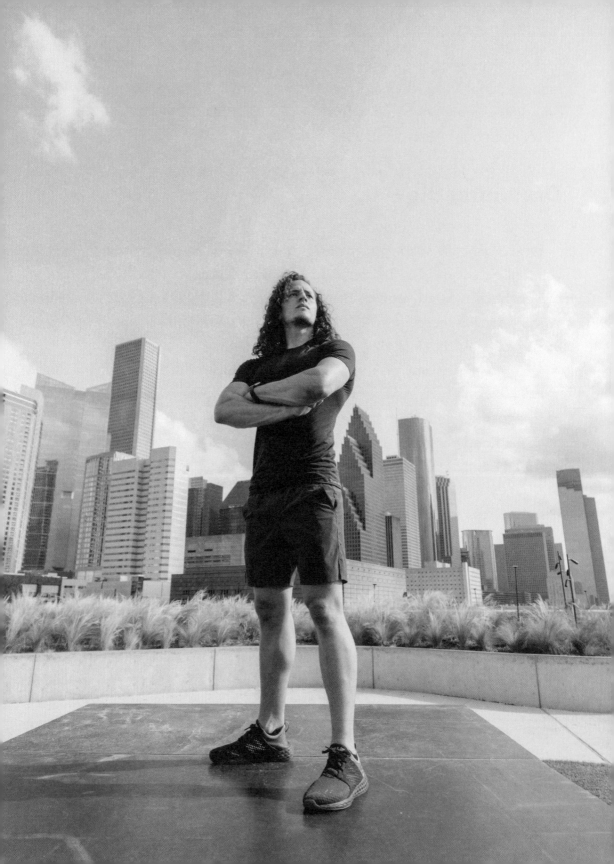

Hospitality

I always go back to my childhood when I think of what a home should be like. Though not perfect, our home was always a safe haven, a place where family and friends could stay if they were traveling or going through a rough patch in life. It was a place where we would share meals, have deep and meaningful conversation together, and of course, play board games and entertain whoever was over that day. A big priority of mine when looking to buy a house is to have guest rooms with multiple beds so we can host people. Growing up, we had several family friends live with us for periods of time—and some cousins who lived with us for years at a time. Our house was known as a safe place for many people, and I thank my parents for making it that way. Anyone could come there and experience the love and kindness of God. The joy of the Lord was always evident, even though my rambunctious ways made our home a little chaotic at times. My parents made it a priority to be the "party" house on the block. We had swing sets, a ropes course, an Air Pogo swinging from a tree, and the largest trampoline we could find—all in the backyard! We had bikes and roller skates, homemade ramps, and first aid kits for the inevitable wipeouts. Our home was where everybody wanted to be.

Both Abby and I grew up in big families, and we see it as a high priority to have the space to be able to host. Eventually, we'd love to raise a big family in a home that we build ourselves on my parents' property, which is on the outskirts of the Houston area.

We've spent years living in a one-bedroom apartment, but even now we're trying to treat it in the same way we'll treat the five-bedroom home we hope to build. We're trying to be faithful with what we currently have so that someday we can be entrusted with more and do on a much larger scale what we already do on a small scale.

Marriage

Nothing has been more exciting and maturing in my life than my marriage to my wife, Abigail. We said our vows and committed our lives to each other before God and men seven years ago. People can pursue personal development and maturity at their own pace, but in marriage, you're in the midst of it 24/7, 365 days a year. The covenant and commitment of marriage brings growth (if you allow it) that nothing else in life can give you.

Abby and I initially met at a mutual friend's going-away party. I believe it's through relationships and community that God helps us to walk with the right people in life. As believers, we trust that God has the right life for us . . . and the right people to walk through life with. Now, we can always mess that up and choose things in life that are different from His best for us, but He can still redirect us because of His mercy and grace. I fully believe that Abigail was hand-selected and orchestrated to be in my life.

I was nineteen years old when a friend told me he was moving. At his party I met a whole bunch of people I'd never known before. They asked what I was

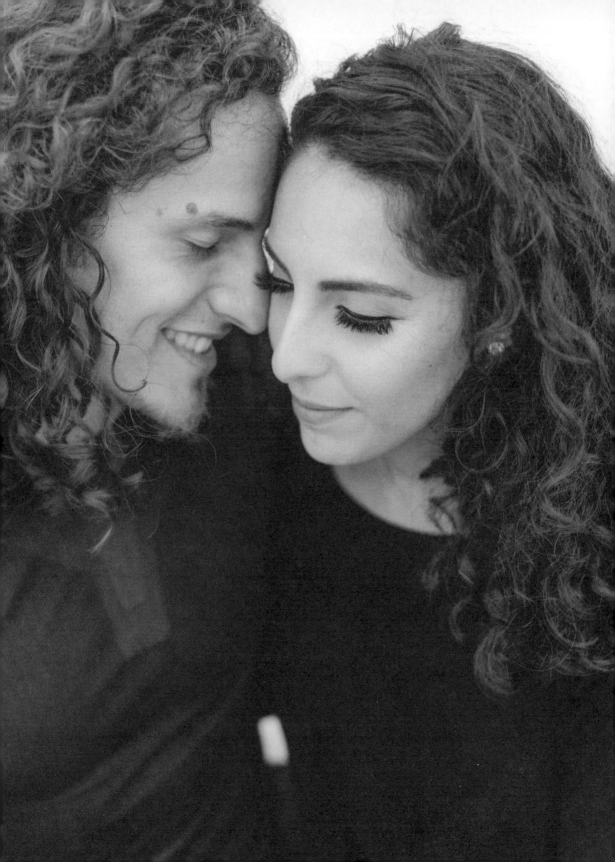

doing after graduating, so I told them I was going to a local school of ministry. And they replied, "Wow, we all go to a school of ministry." How about that! You're right in thinking it was an odd and pretty rare happenstance. But even back then I believed that things happen for a reason. So we talked about the Bible, churches, conferences, pastors, popular worship music, and community. I was glad to make more friends who were on a similar path to mine.

It wasn't until months later that Abby and I started hanging out in group settings. I was in the midst of a relationship with my high school sweetheart when I initially met Abby. So at first I thought Abby was awesome, but I filed her under the "friend" category due to my other relationship.

I was devastated when my high school girlfriend broke up with me. After graduating high school, we both started to change a lot in terms of dreams, goals, and priorities in life. After that relationship ended, I thought, *Lord, I'll never date anyone again unless You bring them across my path.* It was in that new season of singleness that I began to have close friends who were girls in my life again . . . which felt kind of weird after four years of having eyes for only one girl. This new group of friends included Abby, and I liked that a whole lot. If you've met Abby, you know what I'm talking about. I remember thinking, *This girl is really beautiful and really special, and she loves the Lord. Not to mention everything else we have in common, like movies, music, and dreams!*

After months and months of hanging out, we became inseparable—the best of friends, who talked and texted almost every day. She was gorgeous, and she loved overseas missions, loved ministry, and had a passion for life like no one else I had known . . . except me! I finally got the nerve and asked her out . . . only to be rejected several times! She was focused solely on the season of life she was living with God. She was too wise for her own good (or maybe just for what I perceived as my good!). All my cards were on the table about my old relationship. She had never dated anyone before and didn't want to be a rebound for me. We had become the best and most inseparable of friends, and I told her I wanted to see if there was anything there.

"I don't want to feel like a rebound and mess up the friendship," she said. She made it sound so good. But I wanted to be in a more purposeful relationship with her. She said it wasn't a shut door, but simply "not now." In a few months when I asked again, the timing still wasn't right. She was moving to Nashville to help get a ministry on its feet. All of our friends really thought we should date and saw that we could be a great couple together. I thought so too!

I told her that, after coming out of the first relationship, I only wanted to date with the intention of marriage. I had no intention of dating just to date or have fun, contrary to our world's "hookup culture." While we were long distance, she said, "I think I'm ready." And the next time she was in town, I asked her to officially start dating me.

I remember telling her that I had an opportunity to work in this ninja gym and maybe even get on the show one day! Her response was, "Yeah, you and every other guy in the world." After I got into some local competitions and began winning, she started to see that in addition to my abilities, training, and preparation, God might be doing something in that space.

When I first competed on *ANW* and won the qualifiers, she became extremely supportive. Her family (and even my family) initially didn't quite know how big it could become. After dating for almost two years (and saving up little by little for a ring because I already knew I would marry this girl), I went to her parents and said, "Here's the deal . . . I'm head over heels for your daughter, and we're the best of friends. We want to start our life together."

They said, "We like you a lot, but we want to make sure you're able to provide for her. Can you do that?" Through miraculous means, I was able to begin traveling and doing events using my status as a successful athlete on *ANW*. Her parents were happy to give me their blessing when they saw that I was able to provide for their daughter. Abby is also my brand manager and helps me with booking events, which has been a blessing because she is able to travel with me almost everywhere I go!

During that season of pursuing the woman of my dreams, I received two great pieces of advice, which turned into lessons. A close friend of mine said, "Endeavor to love your wife better with each new day." That helps me to always treat my wife as the treasure that she is.

The other piece of advice came from a mentor and spiritual dad of mine who said, "When you say those vows before God and before men—for better or worse, in sickness and health, for richer or poorer—you better mean that. If divorce is *ever* an option, it will inevitably become the only option." So from the get-go, we realized that divorce could never be an option. I've learned sacrificial love, communication, and keeping the bond of unity within our home above all. If Christ sacrificed Himself even unto death for those He loved (all of humanity), then that becomes the standard by which I endeavor to love my own wife, whom I believe God handpicked for me.

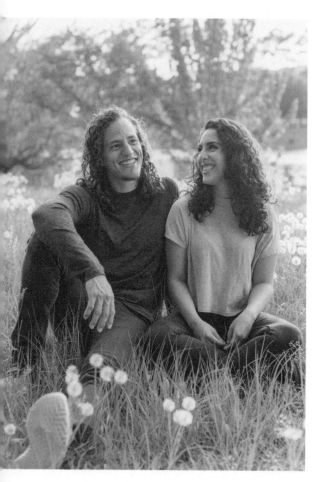

The world wants instant gratification. But in His relationship with the church, the Lord modeled a life of sacrifice for the betterment of the other. The better I love my wife and sacrifice for her my time, energy, and efforts, the more I can see in her eyes that my effort is never wasted, and our relationship continues to blossom and grow over time because of it. Our life together will always show the proof of that commitment.

Mentoring

I began coaching ninjas almost two years before I ever competed on the show, and I've been coaching for almost a decade now. During my years of coaching, I have had the privilege of seeing many students grow and eventually be selected for *American Ninja Warrior Junior*, and now several have also begun competing alongside me on the main show. I'm not old, but these experiences are reminding me that I've been doing this awhile! I'm glad I started when I did, but I sure wish I would have had an opportunity to begin even sooner, not that that was possible at the time. But I trust in the Lord's divine timing and make the most of the time that I'm given.

With the past several years of pandemic shutdown, *Ninja Warrior* put up many precautions regarding the audience (many times opting to not having anyone in the stands), but they did allow "virtual sidelining," where you could watch and cheer on family and friends while they competed. I'm happy to have been able to cheer on my friends and former students during these strange times.

There's joy in seeing the community of ninja warriors reach their potential! It's great to see former students get their shot at the world's toughest obstacle course with a million dollars at stake. Being as competitive as I am, I love having people I know and love step up to the same tier I'm in as an athlete and force me to make sure I'm in top shape! All the techniques and mental tricks I've learned over the years, I teach to them. We all know how devastating it is when we train so hard and then fall. I do my best to give them every advantage I can when they go into competition. There's a real bond in that, a bond that not many people can share.

I don't have to feel threatened by others when I know what I'm capable of and that I've done everything I can to prepare. Ninja isn't a billion-dollar industry, unlike other sports in which athletes sign multimillion-dollar contracts each season. It could easily turn into this huge pressure thing when major contracts are on the line, like in the NFL or NBA. The pressure is *different* in those contexts. I can only imagine.

We're competing on *Ninja Warrior* as more of a passion project, knowing the risks and understanding (sometimes the hard way) that it's a television show. For me, this sport has always been a combination of ministry and pleasure. Yes, it's provided a livelihood for me, but I still give God all the credit for opening up the doors for me to begin doing it in the first place. Again, keep things in perspective.

Seeing young ninjas grow up and excel in the sport is one of the great joys of being a coach. Right now, the first two who come to mind are a brother-and-sister combo, Isaiah and Isabella Wakeham, who have competed on the show for several seasons now. Like me, they are from a home-school family with four kids. They're strong and deeply rooted Christians. These kids are supercool, well-spoken, and self-aware. Isabella has quickly become one of the top females in the sport and still has just begun stepping into her potential as an athlete. She's got the height, the strength, and the mental game down. Both she and Isaiah are *so capable* and have been featured heavily as a brother-sister combo who are incredible competitors and are crushing it.

I can't take credit, but they're two people who have made it into the spotlight after I met them as kids almost a decade ago! They consult with me and several other coaches who compete regularly, asking about courses and different hurdles we've overcome in the mental and physical preparation game. I'm really excited for them and others who are stepping onto the main stage of *Ninja Warrior*! With each new season, the show's producers have upped the difficulty and technicality of the sport, and it's exciting to watch people hit the course! Isaiah and Isabella love the show, they love the sport, and they love competing, but they also see it as a ministry platform, just like I do. There are many other ninjas out there who do the same thing with the platform they have been given.

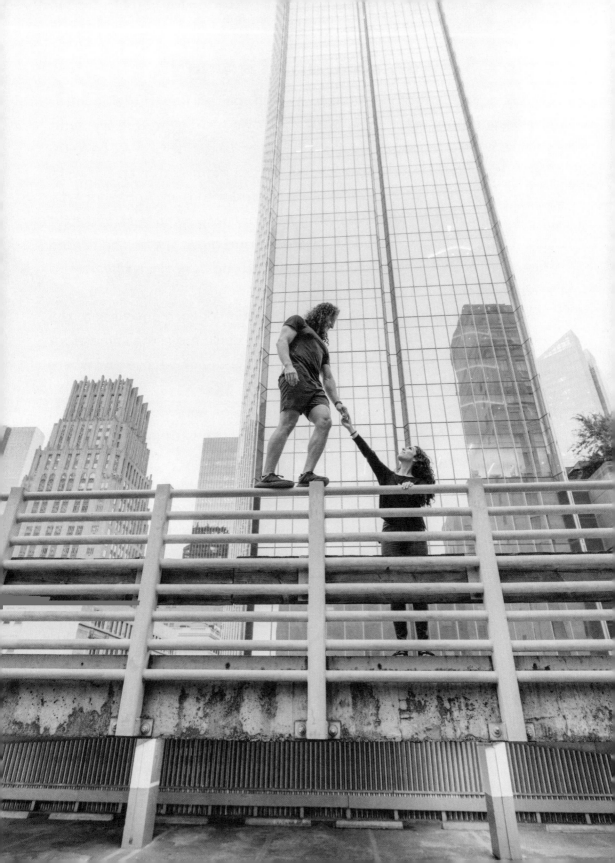

Money, Stewardship, and Tithing

You may wonder what money has to do with spiritual health. Well, a lot!

Everything starts small, like a seed that grows into a great tree over time. If you can handle, manage, and maintain a small amount, God will be faithful in giving you more to work with. We have a promise that as believers, if we're trustworthy with a little, we'll be trusted with a lot. And what type of seed you plant will determine what type of crop you harvest. You start small, work through the setbacks, and learn and grow. There is no reward without risk, and having wise counsel when taking risks always helps with the preparation.

You could say that it's risky to devote a portion of each paycheck to the Lord in the form of a 10 percent tithe. But you could make the same argument about stock investments. It's just a matter of perspective and where your faith is at—or better, who your faith is in.

But I believe that God made me and put me on earth for a reason and a purpose. And one tangible way to show my faith is through my use of money. The Bible says that the *love* of money is the root of all evil, though money itself is not evil. How you think about money simply reveals your heart, regardless of whether you have much or little. If you're stingy with a little, you'll be stingy with a lot. If you're generous with a little, you'll be generous with a lot. If you're careless with a little, you'll be careless with a lot.

I started tithing in high school when I devoted my life to the Lord. Studying the character and nature of God through Scripture, along with His many promises throughout the Bible, made me want to put into practice all I was learning and see its effectiveness in my own life. Proverbs 3:9-10 says to "honor the LORD with your possessions, and with the first-fruits of all your increase; so your barns will be filled with plenty, and your vats will overflow with new wine" (NKJV), and Malachi 3:10 says, "'Bring the whole tithe into the storehouse, that there may be food in my house. Test me in this,' says the LORD Almighty, 'and see if I will not throw open the floodgates of heaven and pour out so much blessing that there will not be room enough to store it'" (NIV). So whether I gave part of a little high school paycheck, or a larger payday from *Ninja Warrior*, I promised to always put God before money.

Part of tithing is putting your money where your mouth is and trusting that God will take care of your needs in every area of your life. And He has *always* taken good care of Abby and me, even when things felt tight or difficult. Some tithes are much larger than others, and one of my annual goals is to see how much I can invest into the Kingdom of God from what He entrusts to me. Abby and I no longer bat an eye at tithing from anything we receive, ninja or otherwise. I don't live solely for money, and I don't work solely for money. I live and work to honor God in all that I do, and money is a by-product of that. I've learned that money makes for a terrible master but a wonderful servant.

We've always said that we didn't want money to control us, so Abby and I continually hold each other accountable in this area as we grow older and life gets more expensive. We are blessed to be a blessing.

If you're a pro in the NFL or NBA, you get paid the big bucks just for showing up. Not so with *ANW*. Money and fame cannot be the motivators because of how difficult the current format is. But honestly, it felt a little bittersweet when I did finally win, because the year prior when I was just a few seconds away from winning, I could have been a grand champion with a million-dollar prize. But winning—even in an expedited season—showed that I've got what it takes and that I can train my body to do what needs to be done while trusting in God to deliver the results.

After winning *ANW* in a year when many people suffered deficits, it was amazing to be able to give a bigger tithe than I've ever been able to give and to honor the Lord with the firstfruits of my increase. The privilege of giving substantially brought a lot of emotions and a newfound confidence that I was on the right path.

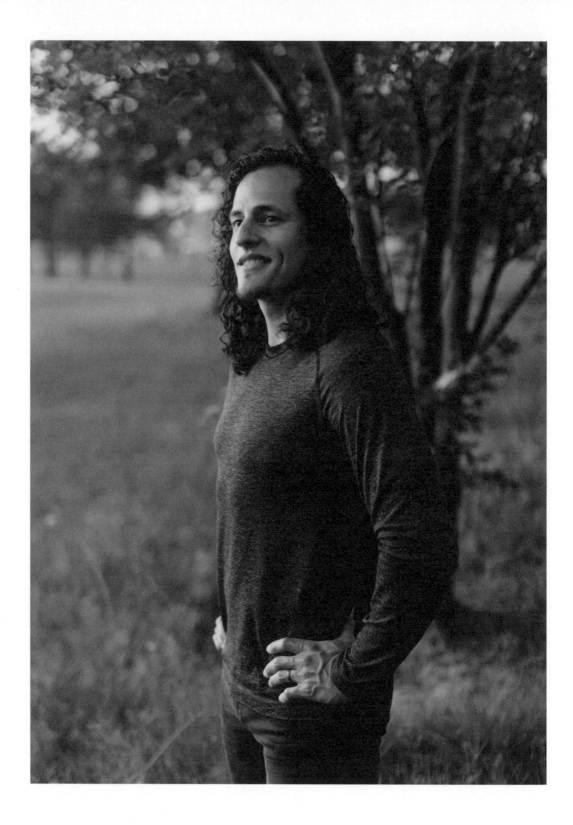

12

LIVING FOR GREATER THINGS

Because of my purpose to be a Christian witness, I feel blessed that people are able to see me deal with adversity in a very public way. Obviously, every athlete competes to win. But as a Christian, I can show that even in defeat, even in an arena where I've given my all and come up mere seconds short, I can honor God with my response to *that* circumstance.

With the lights, cameras, audience, pressure, and new obstacles every year, *anything* can happen, and your season can be over at any moment. In years past on *American Ninja Warrior*, we've seen the strongest athletes go out quickly and unexpectedly because of the smallest break in focus. One of the things I love most about this sport is the laser focus it requires—the way I have to be completely attentive and tune out all of the externals in order to get past an obstacle and through the course. The Christian life is much the same.

Humility is the best possible attitude we can have as athletes and competitors in general, and humility, first and foremost, is born of a robust knowledge of who God is, who I am, and who He has called me to be. *Ninja Warrior* is *the* most humbling sport I've ever been part of because we never know ahead of time exactly what our obstacles are going to be and because we never get a chance to practice them ahead of time. It's rough. Again, it is a lot like life: We have to face unexpected obstacles and learn to navigate them without prior experience.

I recognize that I'm just a human. I know I am created in the image of God, but I am a very imperfect person who will make mistakes, fall, and fail. Ask my wife or anyone in my family. But I will not lose hope. I'll get back up, move forward, and try my hardest to learn from those mistakes and not repeat them. Proverbs 24:16 (NIV) says, "Though the righteous fall seven times," representing many, "they rise again." I will not allow a setback to keep me down. I learned that years ago when I failed Mount Midoriyama and lost a million dollars. I was thinking, *Well, God, I'm disappointed—not in You, but in my results. But Romans 8:28 says that You can work everything together for good for those who love You. Where is the good in this situation?* I really asked myself in that situation, *What is good about losing?*

But as I pondered and prayed about it, I realized that sometimes when we call ourselves Christians and aim for these lofty goals and ideals, failure gives us the chance for even more impact in God's Kingdom than success gives. It's easy to hit a buzzer, get the victory, and lift your hands to give God the glory. Anyone can praise God when they win, and people often do. But it's so much more difficult and will show so much more of a person's faith when they are able to fall and fail and still be thankful. We can still give God glory in spite of how we may feel. We can't let our failures—either in sin or competition—define us. I want to use even failure to encourage and inspire people. My good friend Chris Klimis once said, "We need to be filled with courage, and to do that we need to constantly be encouraged." We need people who genuinely care about us and try to pull the gold out of us. The Bible says that faith comes by hearing, so I love sharing with people all that I've overcome in order to help them in their own struggles.

Life can be difficult at times, which is why I go into each day with many Scriptures that bring encouragement, confidence, and life to me personally. These are Scriptures that I have memorized over the years and pray over myself and my family regularly. This is the fight of faith for me. What's inside

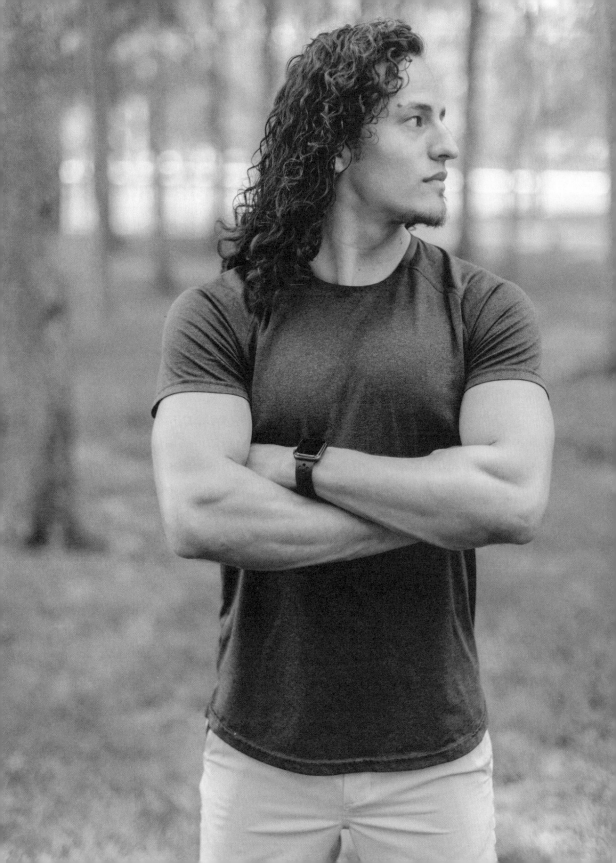

of us is going to be what comes out of us when that pressure hits. If I dwell on my worry and anxiety, then fear and panic will be what comes out of me as a response to that pressure. But I'm reminded that God will never leave us or forsake us (Deuteronomy 31:8), that He has plans to prosper us and not to harm us, and that He will give us a hope and a future (Jeremiah 29:11). I want the truth of the Word of God to come out of me when the pressures of life come against me. That changes the effect of all of life's many valley moments. Even Jesus said, "Here on earth you will have trials and sorrows. But take heart, because I have overcome the world" (John 16:33 NLT).

I'm reminded that Jesus sacrificed His life on the cross to give me freedom and to establish a new covenant. His sacrifice covers my sins not just once but for all time. Jesus now goes before me and comes behind me as a front and rear guard (Isaiah 58:8). God's grace is sufficient for me, and His power is perfected in my weakness (2 Corinthians 12:9).

Personally, I love Matthew 6:27-33 which reads,

> And which of you by being anxious can add a single hour to his span of life? And why are you anxious about clothing? Consider the lilies of the field, how they grow: they neither toil nor spin, yet I tell you, even Solomon in all his glory was not arrayed like one of these. But if God so clothes the grass of the field, which today is alive and tomorrow is thrown into the oven, will he not much more clothe you, O you of little faith? Therefore do not be anxious, saying, "What shall we eat?" or "What shall we drink?" or "What shall we wear?" For the Gentiles [those who aren't walking with the Lord] seek after all these things, and your heavenly Father knows that you need them all. But seek first the kingdom of God and his righteousness, and all these things will be added to you.

The life I'm going to live is one full of faith that God will provide what I need if I love the Lord with all my heart, soul, and mind, and live according to His Word.

Proverbs 3:5-6 says to trust in the Lord with all my heart and lean not on my own understanding, to acknowledge Him in all my ways, trusting that He will make my path straight. My job is to keep God first and trust Him always. He's not shaken and falling off His throne after the years we've just had. Our job is to trust.

I was just seconds away from a million dollars. And I failed. I lost. The next time you lose, just remember you didn't lose a million dollars! After I got out of my feelings and emotions of that whole experience . . . this failure in front of millions of people . . . I asked God how He could use it for good. I've been able to share this message of humility and trust in countless camps, gyms, and churches across the nation.

I've learned that God doesn't view failure the way we view it. Every time I compete, there's the chance that people could see God through me. It reminds me to shine, and shine brightly.

Losing

Having just begun a new decade at 30 years old, I try to keep everything in perspective. As it pertains to *Ninja Warrior*, I remember standing on the starting line the first time, looking around, about to run the course, with a sideline producer ready with the countdown: "3, 2, 1, Go!"—and being terrified. I remember praying, *God, I've trained for this moment my whole life. I'm doing both sports and production right now, which are two things that bring me a lot of joy.* I wanted to show the world how excited and happy I was for that moment right there. Even getting there and getting to compete was a miracle. I prayed, *Okay, God, even if I fall on the first obstacle, I'm going to show the world how grateful I am for this moment right here.*

Losing is never fun. Again, the perspective I try to keep for *Ninja Warrior* is the reality that you can go to ten competitions and get ten different sets of obstacles and have ten different sets of results . . . even rules can vary

ANW SEASON 7: ROULETTE ROW, LAS VEGAS FINALS, STAGE 2, 2015

This was the obstacle that ended my rookie season on *Ninja Warrior* and crushed my hopes and dreams of winning it all my first year. It still irritates me when I think about it! Essentially, the obstacle is two huge upside-down tilted metal baskets that you have to swing around and lache across using your hands. You start on a short runway and trampoline-jump to the first of the two swinging baskets. It's a time-release obstacle, so once you grab onto the first basket you have only a few seconds before you have to jump to the next one; otherwise, you lose your one opportunity. The baskets are so big that if you don't transfer on your first swing, you lose too much momentum and can never get it back again. I remember hitting the trampoline hard but still barely getting my hands on the first basket, which caused my body to be in an arched position. That made me whip around much too fast, and I missed my only chance to make the transfer. My heart sank because I knew what that meant, but I still gave it everything I had because I *needed* to make that transfer in order to move on! I kicked, pulled, and swung with all my might but just couldn't get a big enough swing to make the move. Once I finally dropped (it felt like an eternity), I was so exhausted and pumped in my forearms that I literally had to be pulled out of the water by the crew because I couldn't open my hands or use my arms properly to pull myself out on my own.

After a brief interview with show host Kristine Leahy, I cried tears of frustration and sadness.

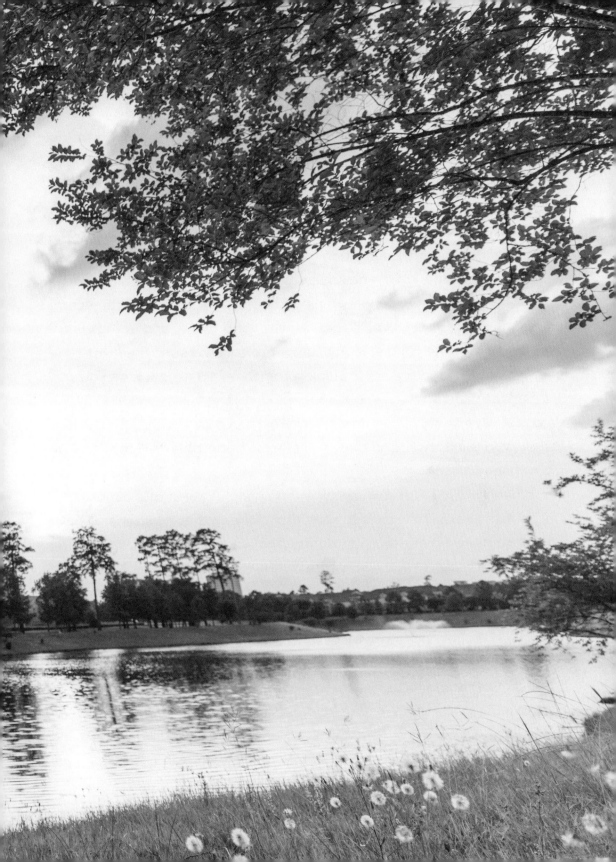

from course to course. No two gyms have identical layouts or competition course designs, but honestly, that's part of the draw for me. It's still so unique in that sense.

I take with a grain of salt the disappointment that comes with falling on a course, because it can happen to anyone, and surprise upsets happen often in this sport. I give ninja competitors a lot of grace because of that, especially outside the TV show at local competitions. Doing this as long as I have, I can look at a course and figure out how I need to hold and move. You get really good at visualization training over time, where you try to see yourself moving through the obstacles before you actually touch them. The better you get at visualization training, the better you'll do on the actual course: how many steps you'll take, moves you'll make, and swings you'll use to navigate the course. Many competitors even count their rest time because some competitions (including the show) limit how long you can rest between obstacles. Use your imagination to the fullest and fill in all the details of what that course run will feel like. Then pray that it actually does feel like you think it will, and above all else, be adaptable and change your plan when necessary.

I've been at a level for a while now where people expect me to make it to the podium or even take the top spot, especially on the show, where I have done it so many times. Recently, during *ANW* season 13, I ended up falling on a qualifiers course for the very first time ever. I was upset with the whole situation . . . I had just won the previous season, but this was a brand-new obstacle I had never touched before, and I was somehow the only person to cause a malfunction on it by getting the ring wedged improperly. Ultimately, it fell back on me for not being more careful with the obstacle. All it takes is one break in focus for you to end up in the water.

Fortunately, the shock and upset of falling for the first time in several years didn't cut me too deeply or last too long, because I still moved on and would have an opportunity at redemption in the semifinals. Pastor Tony

Evans says, "Yesterday's victories will not carry you through today. Neither should yesterday's defeats dominate tomorrow." I wiped the slate clean, focused on my goals, and then crushed the semifinals course. In my opinion, ninja will humble you more than any other sport. Proverbs 16:18 says, "Pride goes before destruction, and haughtiness before a fall" (NLT). Even though falling is inevitable in this sport, I *never* want it to be because of arrogance and oversight on my part. Robert Green Ingersoll said, "The greatest test of courage on earth is to bear defeat without losing heart." In my own experience, that's been proven true time and time again.

I compete to win, and I'm extremely competitive, so I will always give it my all at these events. But in the midst of the competition mentality, there's another strong desire within me, and that's to make time for people and show them love. I'm not just there to perform and showcase my abilities, but to connect with and encourage others—athletes and spectators alike. Because the sport is so community-based, the other side of the coin in competition is ministry. I'll share advice or encouragement when I have opportunity and be a comforting presence to those who may need it later on. It can be a difficult balance at times, but it's always been worth it, and I've never regretted being there for people.

What Does It Mean to Be a Kingdom Ninja?

When you compete on the show, you can't wear branded clothing unless it's your own designs. You won't see guys looking like NASCAR-sponsored racers, decked out in dozens of different brands. I asked myself, *What do I wear? What do I want my legacy to be for the audience? They're going to be seeing me and what I'm wearing. How do I make the most of that opportunity?*

And so I came up with my own brand, Kingdom Ninja. In every city finals episode and beyond, I try to wear a shirt that proclaims a Kingdom core value that I try to live by. Each year I pray about what core value I want to highlight

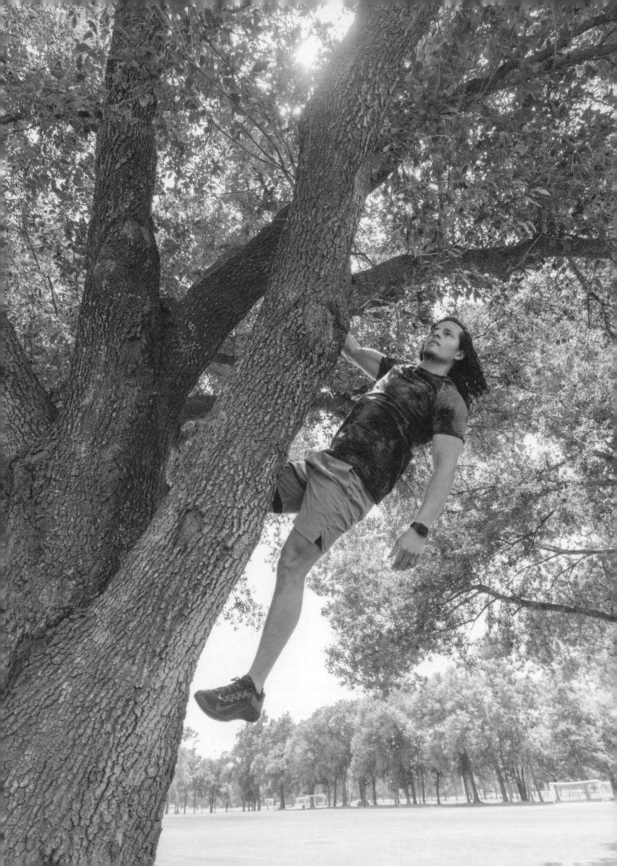

to the millions of others who will be watching that year. Each season I try to wear at least two values. They remind me and the people watching why I am doing what I am doing. I'm trying to make a real impact in the lives of those who are watching me for my fifteen minutes of fame. This is who I am and what I represent. This is what it means for me to be a Kingdom Ninja.

KINGDOM: Each year in the qualifier, I wear "Kingdom" across my chest to show the world that I am a believer—without being cheesy or appearing to shove my faith down anyone's throat. I wear it in remembrance of Matthew 6:33, that my priorities are to "seek first the kingdom of God" and live righteously.

HONOR: I chose to wear "Honor" across my chest as a reminder to be a man of honor. I love the Japanese culture of honor toward family and country, but also—biblically speaking—honor is like currency to God because honor always led to miracles and revelation. I love that.

ALIVE: I chose to wear "Alive" on my shirt to share the testimony of my life and to show that what was currently unfolding with my ninja career came after being made fully alive in Christ and pursuing a relationship with Him.

GLORY: I chose to wear "Glory" across my shirt to showcase to the world that I'm living my life for the glory of God in all things I do, ninja and otherwise.

HOPE: I chose to wear "Hope" across my chest because I understand that people gain hope from watching the show, hearing the stories of how the ninjas have overcome various life challenges and physical obstacles. But more importantly, I wore "Hope" on my shirt to point the world to the saving hope that is found in Jesus.

LEGACY: I chose to wear "Legacy" across my chest because I want my life to leave an impact and legacy—not just by competing on *American Ninja Warrior* but also through my family, friends, and all who will be affected by my life. I make decisions based on a legacy that will last for generations (Acts 13:36).

COMMUNITY: I chose to wear "Community" across my chest during the lockdown and pandemic year to shine a light on the need for each of us to have people in our lives who truly love and care for us, even if not perfectly. We were never meant to live as lone wolves. We all need community. Certain people are like pillars in my life: family, friends, and leaders who sharpen me as iron sharpens iron, watch over me like mothers and fathers do, and help keep me on the path I believe the Lord is leading me on. My Pastor Randy Needham says, "Find your family, find your destiny." That has been so true for me in my life, and I'm grateful to be part of my community. Make sure that you are walking in community.

SACRIFICE: I chose to wear "Sacrifice" across my chest because in life we all must make sacrifices: for our family, for our dreams, and for our futures. Most importantly, I wore it to acknowledge the ultimate sacrifice that was made on the cross of Calvary. The greater the sacrifice, the greater the reward.

REDEMPTION: I chose to wear "Redemption" across my chest for various reasons. First, in one respect, it was because I had fallen for the first time in my career on a qualifier course, and I wanted redemption going into the semifinals. More importantly though, I wore it as a reminder that in this life we can find redemption through Jesus. I am redeemed though imperfect. I am forgiven though I fall and fail. My past does not dictate my future . . . all because of who my faith is in. If the Son sets you free, you will be free indeed (John 8:36).

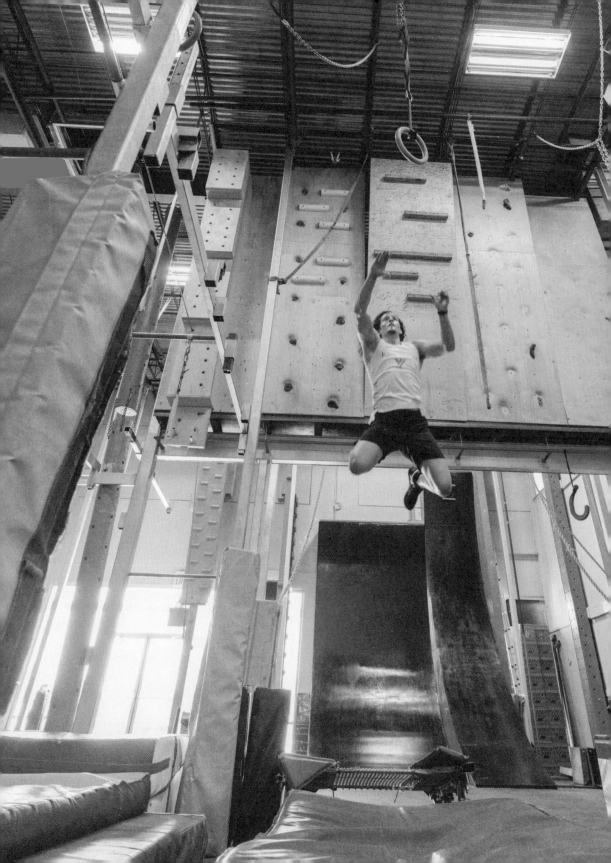

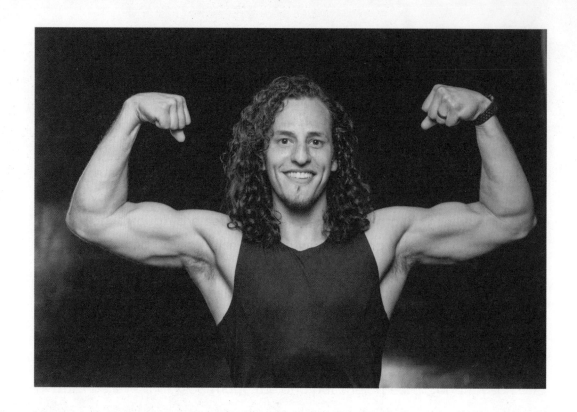

ABOUT THE AUTHOR

Daniel Gil is an *American Ninja Warrior* athlete, the 2020 *ANW* Champion, and a seven-time national finalist. He is also a motivational speaker, a worship leader, and a ninja OCR trainer. He and his wife, Abby, live in Houston, Texas.

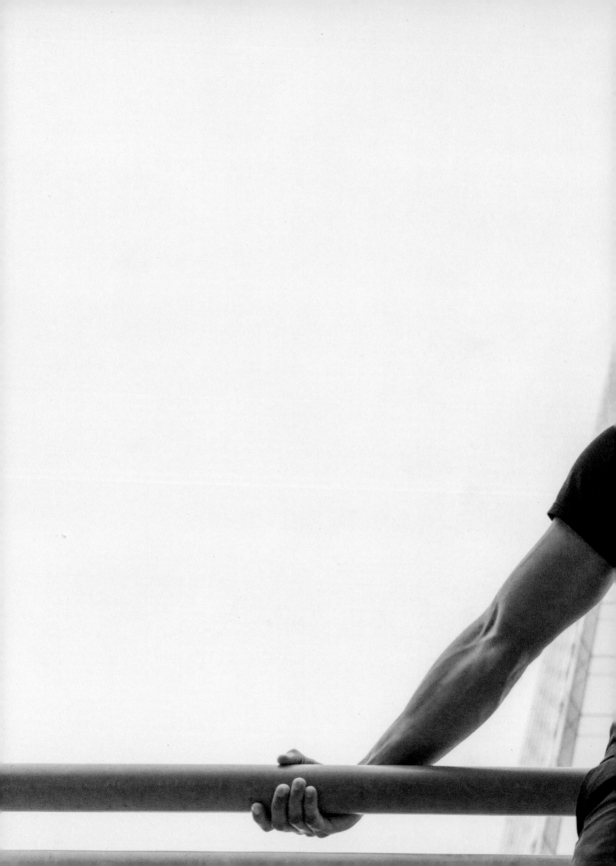